How to Become
A Successful Personal
Trainer

Chris Hitchko CSCS

Contents

Preface

You're about to embark on one of the best decisions of your life - to become a personal trainer. There are few professions where you can wake up and truly be excited to do what you're passionate about. Your office will be filled with weights, high energy, personal records, blood, sweat, and tears. I've been a personal trainer for over 10-years and there's nowhere else I'd rather be. I love pushing people out of their comfort zones and would like to augment your journey toward becoming a successful personal trainer!

I'd like to thank everyone who helped make this book come to fruition. If we continue to focus on the great in this industry via educating the next generation, we will continue to make giant strides in this new industry. Thank y'all for helping make this book a reality.

Matt Benson for helping me gather my thoughts and construct something tangible. You're an incredible editor, even better writer, and great friend (I still want to cut your face off.)

Tony Gentilcore for being one of the kindest strength coaches I've met. There are few more humble and brilliant strength coaches in the world. You're going to be a great dad!

Bret Contreras for putting up with my quasi stalker tendencies.

The Show Up Fitness Academy Board of Education. We will change the entry standards for becoming a personal trainer while spreading the good 'ol word of science.

The trainers at Show Up Fitness Santa Monica & Dublin for being the best personal trainers I've ever worked with.

Jamie Verab you're a great athlete, graphic designer (100% his idea for this badass cover), entrepreneur, and friend. You've helped me get out of the comfort zone ever since our days at UCONN, and we will be at the top together.

The Hitchko family for being my support system. When in doubt, y'all have had my back when others said it wasn't possible. Coulda, woulda, shoulda; I'm proud to say, "I'VE SHOWN UP!"

Jackson Foy. For being the best hunting buddy anyone could ever ask for. "Hey, was that a chucker?"

Show Up Fitness will be known as the premier personal training company who redefined the personal training industry.

So, without further ado…

Introduction

Are you tired of being miserable at your soul-sucking 9–5?

Are you tired of devoting 40 hours per week to an unfulfilling, meaningless job that slowly morphs you into a shapeless blob-like Jabba the Hutt instead of the Gisele Bündchen/Tom Brady living inside you?

Are you tired of compromising your happiness?

Are you going to settle for mediocrity, or do you want to change lives?

My name is Chris Hitchko, a personal trainer with 12 years of experience and owner of Show Up Fitness, an exclusive personal training gym with two locations in Santa Monica, CA, and Dublin, CA. I've trained thousands of clients, I've taught over 700 personal trainers, and my business is growing at a rate so fast I can barely keep up. I truly love what I do. I'm my own boss, I've written two books (with two more coming out soon), I bench pressed 315 last year, I live by the beach, and I work around 40 hours a week.

I know this probably sounds great (and it is—I've never been happier in my life), but it wasn't easy to get there. I credit my success to persistence, hard work, and SHOWING UP ever since I began training in 2006. Am I the best? Not even close. But I've surrounded myself with legendary trainers—trainers like Dan John, Tony Gentilcore, Bret Contreras, Ben Bruno, Nick Tumminello, Kellie Davies, Eric Cressey, Dean Somersey, Molly Galbraith, John Rusin, Tim Henriques, Alwyn and Rachel Cosgrove, and Sohee Lee—who are all smarter, stronger, and better coaches than I am.

That's what you're getting with this book, the wealth of knowledge I've accumulated through my own personal experience and from learning from the best. I've read hundreds of books, taken countless courses, and made more mistakes than I care to admit. But now, after thousands of personal training sessions and over 700 personal trainers graduated, I can say that, even though I might not be the absolute best, I'm definitely among the more knowledgeable people in the industry. I wrote this book because I want to impart all that knowledge to you. I want to help you avoid all the mistakes I made and the misconceptions I carried with me for far too long. I want you to start your personal training career with eyes wide open.

My journey into the fitness world began when I was in fourth grade. My dad was a fitness enthusiast and my parents gave me and my three brothers two after-school options: do your homework, or go to the gym with Dad. I wanted to get stronger for Basketball and Track, so while other kids were playing video games, I was reading every fitness magazine I could get my hands on, or I was in the gym lifting—probably a lot like you. After graduating in 2006 with a degree in Kinesiology, I was hired as a personal trainer at Bladium, a 10,000-square-foot globo-gym featuring two indoor soccer fields, a rock climbing wall, and a restaurant. My first year of training sucked because I didn't have any money, had zero guidance, and I never trained a celebrity or athlete—WTF! The reality vs. expectations brought me down to earth. I had split shifts at two different gyms: 6 a.m.–12 p.m. at one gym, and 3 p.m.–8 p.m. at the other, five days a week. That was my schedule for my first four years. I would usually train a client or two every weekend, so time off was a rarity, and my paychecks were like Justin Bieber's biceps—SMALL. (If only I had his bank account!) When I began teaching, I taught for 44 hours, trained regularly, and worked every Saturday that I can remember. I came to realize that my clientele base as a personal trainer is more typically a morbidly obese version of your most annoying aunt or uncle.

Where were all the superstar athletes, models, and actors the industry had led me to believe I was going to be training? Nowhere to be found.

I remember my first personal training assessment in 2006, Mrs. Williams. These 60-minute assessments are designed to show the value in working with a personal trainer. Properly administered, the client should see the value in training with you, because you've reviewed goals, asked open-ended questions, and analyzed their movement. During my first assessment with Mrs. Williams, I talked to her the entire time, didn't ask any open-ended questions, and discussed the how the quadriceps are made up of the vastus lateralis, medialis, intermedius, and rectus femoris… SHE DIDN'T CARE! I learned from the experience, but if I had this book at the time, I could have potentially signed her up as a client instead of scaring her away with all the esoteric science jargon. If I could go back and give myself advice, I'd say wake up every day at 5 a.m., read more books, network with personal trainers, start a book club, go to workshops, smile more, stop running, get out of your comfort zone, take more classes, and learn to Deadlift, Squat, and Bench Press.

This isn't a book on how to get clients, or a shortcut to becoming a celebrity trainer. It's an honest approach on what to expect if you're thinking of becoming a personal trainer, or if you've been recently certified.

Roadmap to
How To Become A Successful Personal Trainer:

Τhe Truth About the Personal Training Industry—Certifications vs. Education

The Average Day in the Life of a Trainer (Business Aspects of Becoming a Personal Trainer)

How to Get Interviewed and Hired at a Corporate Gym (Equinox/Crunch/24 Hour Fitness)

How to Make 75k as a Personal Trainer (The Benchmark for Happiness)

Interviews from Top Personal Trainers

I've interviewed my most successful students and colleagues to help educate you on how to become a successful trainer without making the same mistakes I did. I'm going to be transparent so there's no ambiguity or confusion about the personal training industry. Social Media exacerbates the personal training myths, like it's a magical job that doesn't require you to work, and is all about posting hot selfies in front of a mirror at the gym. In reality, clients cancel all the time, go on vacations, disappear, and in some respects, can be just as annoying as customers in the 9–5 world. As a personal trainer, you only get paid when you render a personal training session, so if you're making four grand a month training 100 sessions, what do you think will happen during Christmas vacation? That's right—you're going hungry unless you've planned ahead. If you do not prepare for situations like this, you'll lose your passion quickly, and your personal training career will come to an end before you know it.

THE COLD HARD TRUTH

I spent years as an idealistic, ambitious young trainer, dedicated to nothing except helping my clients fulfill their goals and gaining as much knowledge as I possibly could. This wasn't necessarily a bad thing, because my head and heart were in the right place, but I was naïve. Eventually, after training thousands of clients, learning more about the industry, and studying the habits of other trainers around me, I realized there are two fundamental truths about the personal training industry:

1- Most personal trainers are idiots.

2- The industry is a clusterfuck.

And the two are related.

If any trainer is offended by me saying that most personal trainers are idiots, it's because they're one of the idiots. Most trainers take a simple certification test like the National Exercise & Sports Trainers Association (NESTA) and the Aerobics and Fitness Association of America (AFAA), and hope to end up selling treadmills or diet products on TV (here's looking at you, Jillian Michaels!).

The most popular certification is the National Academy of Sports Medicine (NASM), which is one of the most highly regarded certifications in the corporate gym industry. When I graduated college in 2006, I was informed I needed to get my NASM certification, despite having a kinesiology degree, and spending a year in one of the top kinesiology programs in the country (UCONN). I also had arguably the most respected certification (American College of Sports Medicine), but apparently that wasn't good enough to start training clients—I needed my NASM certification. At the time, I thought maybe this NASM certification was the real deal, and maybe I didn't know anything after my four years of college and the American College of Sports Medicine certification. I started to question everything I knew.

Was the NASM some magical new test that was going to expose gaps in my knowledge?

Advanced anatomy with insertion points and muscular actions?

In-depth programming?

A practical interview by top Exercise Physiologists?

Nope. None of those.

It turns out, the NASM test—the most sought after certification—cost $600 and took less than one month of half-assed study. For shits and giggles, I recently took the NASM test again to see if it's changed. I passed it in 22 minutes. It's a joke. I found it appalling that something as dynamic and complex as the biomechanics of human movement should be reduced to such a bullshit certification.

I'm sorry to get your panties in a bundle if you had some vague illusions about the personal training industry being "super professional" and "highly regulated," but most trainers take a simple certification, pass it by studying themselves, and then train people how they like to train. Once I realized this, I was shocked. If you want to become a doctor, you need an undergraduate degree, pass the MCAT's, and then be accepted and attend medical school. To become a lawyer, you need to get a degree, pass the LSAT, earn your Juris Doctor degree (JD), and then pass the state Bar Examination. To be a Certified General Electrician, you need an apprenticeship of 8,000 hours with work experience and at least two years of school to be considered to take the state test. There are a lot of "professional trainers" (aka dipshits) putting their clients' health at risk and pretending to know what they're doing, when all they did was pass that very simple test.

Can you blame them? How many careers do you know where you can take a $600 test and then begin charging between $50 and $75 per hour? The problem with the personal training industry is that there's no uniform schooling process. NESTA, AFAA, NASM…there are many different personal training certifications you can take, and *the most highly regarded of them all is a joke. So* most personal trainers are idiots *because* the industry is a clusterfuck. See what I mean?

Fortunately, most personal trainers who pay their $600 and venture out into the personal training world end up failing, but unfortunately, this sets up most trainers, as well as their clients, for failure.

Here's the path to becoming a typical (failing) personal trainer:

Name: Shrek

Find a certification that is approved by The National Commission for Certifying Agencies (NCCA).

Purchase the material for the certification that you choose—usually the cheapest and easiest to pass. Expect to spend between $100 and $500 to take the test and get the textbook.

Receive material in the mail one week later or immediately if you can study online.

Begin reading the material.

Start reading forums on how people passed the certification.

Begin to take as many sample tests as you can.

Barely read the text because people tell you to focus on certain topics.

Schedule the exam a month after you received the material.

Pass the one-to-two-hour certification.

Boom! Shrek is a certified personal trainer.

The problem with Shrek is that he has no idea about how to actually train people and that is the scariest part. Shrek is going to train your friends and family.

Does Shrek understand anatomy and human movement? No.

Does Shrek understand how personal training affects basic injuries? No.

Does Shrek understand biochemistry and nutrition? Nope.

What about programming and periodization? NO WAY.

Shrek will train people as he trains himself. The worst part is that Shrek is not only a horrible personal trainer; he also has no idea about how to sell his services. He doesn't even understand the business. This means that his approach to training is based on fear tactics, so if you're his client, he'll show you exercises that will make you uncomfortable and if you protest, he'll persist that pain equals gain, and that's why you need to train with him. After you waste hundreds of dollars and countless hours with him, you'll think about quitting. Shrek will blame your lack of results on your diet and lead you to believe you need to eat less and do more cardio. Maybe you purchase another training package, but the results will be the same. Blame on you, but no shame on Shrek!

Once I realized (and became frustrated with) the clusterfuck world of personal training, I wanted to be part of positive change in the industry, so I decided to start teaching prospective personal trainers. I was hired by The National Personal Training Institute (NPTI) in 2009, taught there for over seven years, and graduated 100's of successful trainers. While I ensured each of my student trainers understood the basic mechanics of personal training and were knowledgeable on all aspects of personal training, I still felt there was a void. I wanted each student to have a comprehensive education, encompassing all aspects of personal training—the mechanics of an individual training session, the realities of the industry, the business, and the lifestyle of hard work required to succeed. I left NPTI in 2016 with the goal of redefining the personal training industry entry standards. NPTI required the instructors to teach the NASM curriculum (some locations teach from other textbooks, but where I was teaching it was strictly NASM). Teaching NASM was like sitting on a cactus to scratch your ass—very unpleasant but a means to an end. Plus, I knew that my vision of changing the personal training industry wasn't going to happen teaching NASM.

That's why I created my own school, **The Show Up Fitness Personal Training Academy.** My academy is a four-month, 500-hour course, which allows you to gain experience training real people, with an education that persists throughout the course of your career. The Academy will have its own diploma, which is recognized nationwide as a premier personal training school. At **Show**

Up Fitness Academy, future trainers learn anatomy, physiology, nutrition, biomechanics, AND intern at Show Up Fitness in Santa Monica. During these months, you'll shadow seasoned personal trainers, write programs, learn how to develop a business plan, work out daily, have mock interviews with management at Equinox, teach small group classes, and train clients one-on-one. You'll have floor hours like at Equinox or Crunch. At the end of the four months, you'll have to pass a 150-question exam and practical. The practical portion will consist of writing out a program and training a client while being observed. Another unique aspect is our Board of Education. I have a medical doctor, PhD in Nutrition, Exercise Physiology, and Doctorate of Physical Therapy whom I consult with. I'm the lead instructor, but I'm teaching the science of movement, not indoctrination. A problem I saw with most certifications is that they teach you their doctrine and want you to drink their punch. Every trainer I've taught, I strongly preach, "When you graduate, you'll be a trainer who can think for themselves, not a NASM or 'Cert ABC' Trainer. Not at the Academy. I'm like Frodo from *Lord of the Rings*, and with my Board of Education, *we're* The Fellowship—NERD!"

You'll be a successful personal trainer if you follow these steps and implement the advice from those who've been in the trenches for decades. Most importantly, you need to remember why you originally got into this field: *to help people* (not to post selfies of your glutes or abs on Instagram). Stop thinking about yourself for once, or how many "likes" you've recently got with your shirtless gym photo. Instead, concentrate on helping those who are struggling to lose fat, move without pain, press or pull more weight, and look their best. The moment you lose track of helping other people, that's when you're doomed. Start with this eBook, and finish with the **Show Up Fitness Personal Training Academy.**

What's the Difference between an Education and Certification?

The first change I'd make to the personal training industry is entry standards. Amongst other professions, we're looked at as a joke, and I understand why. An at-home study kit and then a two-hour test to be considered a professional in fitness? Get out of here! I believe change begins by educating the masses. So, what's the difference between a certification and an education?

The idea of certifications is that they measure the ability to apply knowledge and skills in the role of a professional. Passing a certification should establish that you're *minimally competent*. It doesn't mean you know everything required to be considered an expert. Education is foundational knowledge and skills, measuring the ability to retain information, and it encompasses as broad a swath of information as you'd like. I have no doubt that many of you can sit at home and, with enough study, probably have what it takes to pass the NASM certification. But what I provide at the **Show Up Fitness Training Academy** is an *Education*, not just the tools to be minimally competent. I'm so confident in the services I provide that I teach monthly prep courses to pass the NASM certification. I do this at no cost to the students, and when I compare the students attending the **Show Up Fitness Personal Training Academy** versus those who are studying at home, not surprisingly, the difference is frightening. Like a student of mine once said, "The reason I decided to come to school is because I can't ask the book a question. When I'm in class with you, if I don't understand something, I can ask you to explain it."

Usually, if a student doesn't understand something, they'll skip that topic and hope they're not tested on it. Don't get me wrong—I'm not saying if you've passed NASM and only NASM that you're guaranteed to be an idiot. There are trainers who've taken these certifications and done well—it's just rare. The few that do well are good about continuing their education after they become certified.

What Are the Best Certifications?

Until the Show Up Academy gets approved for our own diploma, you'll have to settle for a lesser-than certification. So among the 200+ not-so-great options, which ones are the best?

The top three tiered certifications (in order of most challenging and respectable):

1- NSCA,

2- ACSM,

3- NASM.

NSCA-CPT

The National Strength and Conditioning Association, is a non-profit organization. They have one of the top journals of science, the *Journal of Strength and Conditioning Research*—JSCR. When you see the word "journal," it's not what Becky and Sam are using to write down their thoughts. A journal is a monthly or quarterly publication intended to progress science with the newest studies. The NSCA has the Certified Personal Training (CPT) and Certified Strength and Conditioning Specialist (CSCS) exam. The CPT is a 155-question exam geared to work with athletes. You need to be 18 years of age and currently CPR/AED certified. The majority of the exam is based off of assessments, programming, and proper exercise technique. The CPT is a tad bit easier than the ACSM-CPT, but still very challenging. The price for the CPT is around $400.

NSCA-CSCS

If you want to work with collegiate or professional athletes, you should consider the CSCS. This is considered by many to be the Gold Standard within the certifications because you need a college degree. The CSCS is a 4-hour, 200+ question exam with a scientific portion and video analysis. I was impressed with the scientific questions that were asked and the athlete profiling. You need to know what's a good 40-time, vertical jump, bench press, and squat for Division 1 male and female athletes. One negative aspect to the CSCS is that the degree doesn't need to be science related. Weird, right? The CSCS examination is very challenging. I failed one portion and had to re-take it. The price for the CPT is around $475.

ACSM

The American College of Sports Medicine is a non-profit organization. The exam is 115 questions long. You need to be 18 years of age and currently CPR/AED certified. The questions are pretty evenly distributed across the board in client assessments, programming, legal, business, and advertising. The big emphasis is around Coronary Artery Disease Risk Stratifications—e.g., how many risks does a client have if they have a blood pressure of 135/88 mm Hg, BMI of 31, exercises three times a week for 30 minutes for the previous 2 months, and their mother had a heart attack at age 62? What's their risk stratification? The ACSM is for individuals who want to work in a clinic with exercise physiologists addressing disease. In my opinion, I felt like this was the most challenging exam. The price is around $400.

NASM

The National Academy of Sports Medicine is a profit organization. Dr. Clark is a top Physical Therapist, aiming to fix the obesity epidemic by identifying overactive and underactive muscles within the Human Movement System, which is currently being debunked. The exam has 120 questions and you need to be 18 years of age and currently CPR/AED certified. As a profit organization, NASM has numerous tests that you can pay to take, e.g. CES, PES, FNS, WLS (these each cost between $300 and $500). These exams are taken at home, with an open book (or have someone smart with you to help you take it, they'll never know), and then you'll attain the title of a "Specialist." The CPT is bias towards the OPT model (Optimal Performance Training) and the acute variables within. When I took this exam, I felt they focused more on business development over scientific principles like anatomy. In my opinion, this was the easiest of the three exams. The price is around $500.

If you want to be a respected personal trainer, go to a school that spends at least 300 hours in a classroom, learning proper exercise technique, nutrition, practical aspects, and business development. In other words, go to a school that actually *educates* you on the business of being a successful personal trainer. If you must get a certification, I would suggest getting the ACSM or NSCA-CPT. As a gym owner, and hiring manager at gyms, I would think twice about hiring a NASM trainer or any other trainer unless they could get 8/10 on this quiz:

1. Circle the 17 muscles that comprise the shoulder, the Rotator Cuff Muscles:

Teres Major   Brachialis   Bicep Femoris
        Tricep Brachii

Vastus Lateralis   Serratus Anterior   Supraspinatus
        Erector Spinae

Pectoralis Minor Bicep Brachii   Trapezius Minor Levator Major

Teres Minor   Subspinatus   Infraspinatus
        Semitendinosis

Rectus Femoris   Deltoid   Anterior Tibilais Levator
Scapula

Coracobrachialis   Subscapularis   Latissimus   Dorsi
        Sternocleidomastoid

Scalenes   Rhomboid Minor   Trapezius   Levator
Minor

Pectoralis Major Soleus   Rhomboid   Major
        Brachioradialis

Gastrocnemius   Peroneals   Temporal   Minor
        Deltidus Minimus

2. Name the agonist, antagonist, synergist and stabilizers during a bench press? Military press? Squat? Pull-up?

3. What are the four ligaments that make up the knee? (Abbreviations are ok.)

4. What are the patterns of human movement?

5. What are the six nutrients?

6. What is Basal Metabolic Rate? What is Thermal Effect of Food? What is NEAT (Non-Exercise Activity Thermogenesis)?

7. Design a workout for this client: Amber, 37 years old, 169lbs, who hasn't worked out in 5 years. Write out reps/sets/rest & regressions/progressions for each movement.

8. Draw and label the Size Principle. Explain the difference between Type I & Type II muscle fibers?

9. What is creatine?

10. What is the difference between the ATP-PC system and aerobic metabolism?

Bottom Line: Go to school to learn how to become a personal trainer; don't settle for the easy way out by taking a 100-question exam.

How to Become a Successful Personal Trainer

As you can see, there's a big difference between education and certification. You need a certification to start training, but you need an education to succeed in the long term. The **Show Up Fitness Academy** offers education that sets you up for success, and my philosophy for developing students into successful person trainers can be described using the Acronym H.E.L.P. N.I.C.K (see below), as well as all the lessons I've learned from the most successful personal trainers and their mentality for success. Those lessons I've broken down into what I call "the checklist to be a successful personal trainer."

H.E.L.P. N.I.C.K.

I don't know about you, but when I croak, I don't want to be remembered as average. I want to be known as significant. Why settle for mediocrity? To quote one of the best trainers of all time:

"Do, or do not. There's no try."

–Yoda.

This goes with everything in life. If you want the pretty girl or handsome guy, the pay raise, or a better house, GO AND GET IT! If you're wavering from your goals or don't feel like you're on the right path, just remember the acronym H.E.L.P. N.I.C.K., and you'll get pointed back in the right direction.

HUNGER

To be successful, you first have to have the hunger to succeed. Motivational Speaker Eric Thomas gives the following example:

A mentor and his mentee are looking at the ocean. The mentor asks, "How badly do you want it?" The mentee says, "I want it BAD!" The mentor looks over at him and nods to follow him into the water. He follows. As the water gets up to shoulder level, the mentor looks over and says, "How bad?" The mentee replies, "More than you know it!" The mentor grabs him and forces him underneath the water. He continues to hold him under until his last breath is almost up, and then he releases. The mentor looks at the mentee and says, "You need to want it as bad as you wanted that last breath."

You have to be that hungry, and it has to reflect everything you do in your career. Posting on IG that you're "GRINDING", "HUSTLING", or an "ENTREPRENEUR" usually means you're trying to be an Instagram celebrity, not a successful personal trainer. I don't want to hear about your grind, I want to see it with your success stories. You need to be willing to take on any and every opportunity to train people. The hunger to be significant should never leave your bones.

ENERGY

Most of your clients will not enjoy their jobs. They're coming to you because you're a motivator. As the very successful personal trainer Martin Rooney says, "Make your enthusiasm for success stronger than your fear of failure and you will become unstoppable." When client #1 walks into the door at 5 a.m., you need to bring 110% of everything you have. You better be smiling, happy, and at the top of your game, because that's what they signed up for. Imagine getting yelled at by your boss, wife, husband, or shareholders for 90% of your day. The last thing a client wants to think about is life problems outside of the gym; they SHOWED UP to get an amazing workout. When the session is over, you want them to be so fired up that they're going to go tell ten other people how badass of a trainer you are. Clients will look forward to each session because of your energy. When client #10 walks in at 9 p.m., your energy still needs to be 110%—no excuses. Leave all your bullshit at the door and focus on helping your clients reach their goals. Get your pompoms out because it's your time to razzle dazzle baby—BRING THAT ENERY!

Looks

Would you go to a dentist who was missing teeth? I don't think so. You have to be a walking billboard of your services. Being a personal trainer is superficial, there's no other way around it. Our clients want to look better naked, and if you don't look the part, how can you expect them to believe you're the one to help. Practice what you preach. You don't need to be a bikini competitor or The Hulk, but I always want a prospective client to look at me and say, "I want his body. He must be a trainer."

Also, looking the part doesn't only apply to superficial aesthetics. You need to be professional. That means not cussing like a drunken sailor, being on time with a smile on your face, smelling like a fresh garden of roses (not like a hobo on the subway), and having a sturdy handshake. I don't know about you, but I'm going to let my physique speak for itself—Show Up, or Shut Up.

Personality

The best, most successful personal trainers are friendly and sociable. If you can't relate to people, you're going to have a difficult time as a trainer. Being able to adapt to various clients is key. Be a chameleon and have common sense. Don't discuss religion or politics, and if you do, take the side of the clients. I recently had a client who loved Trump. Me: "Yaaa Trump!" Later in the same day, I had a client who hated Trump. Me: "Trump is an idiot!" Political and religious differences will only lead to arguments and the potential loss of a client. Approach your personal training sessions the same way you would approach Thanksgiving dinner with your future in-laws. Don't argue just because you feel passionately about some political or religious view. You're there to train clients, not to debate the comprehensive immigration reform or whether the Bible should be taken literally.

I challenge students to be able to go up to a person at Starbucks and begin a conversation around exercise and nutrition. You need to be able to spark a conversation with anyone and not have any fear. Smile, be ingenious, and don't be a creep. Having an outgoing personality can get you very far in the training world.

Again, don't be a creep.

Networker

Do you know many personal trainers? I live in Santa Monica and I've been told it's the largest per-capita personal-trainer-to-person ratio in the world. Everyone and their grandpa seems to be a personal trainer, so what separates you from the much more ripped Todd, or prettier Jessica? You need to impress people to the point where you're the first person that comes to mind when they think about who they'd like to train with. I guarantee you that your hair stylist, barista, and best friend can name at least five personal trainers. Why would they recommend you over another trainer?

Find a maven. A maven is someone who's highly connected. We all know that guy at the gym who knows everyone, or the regular at the bar who tips very well. These are the kinds of people that you need to train FOR FREE. If you're not training 30 hours a week, you need to fill those empty slots with mavens: Bar tenders, barbers, tattoo artists, secretaries, personal assistants, and dog walkers. Transform their bodies, and they'll do the rest. The average person works 40 hours a week. If you don't have solid clientele base, start training for free. With that being said, don't offer it for "free." The conversation should sound something like this,

"Mr. Barista at Starbucks. I'm a trainer and I would like to train you. My rates are normally $75/hour, but I'll train you for free. Here's the deal. You HAVE TO WIN THE WEEK. That means workout 4x with weights, write me a Yelp AND Google review, and I'm going to track your transformation progress with before and after photos. At the end of the three months, if you refer me two clients, I'll continue to train you for free. How does this sound?"

Make it worth their while and they'll SHOW UP!

At the local Equinox, 60% of members check-in and go straight to an aerobics class. How many classes have you taken? As a new trainer, your goal should be to take every class on the schedule at least three times. Introduce yourself to the instructor, offer to train them for free, and ask if they'd be kind enough to let the class know that there's a trainer present in the class today. Smile, work hard, motivate others, and introduce yourself to the people around you. Classes are a comfort zone; dumbbells and the weights areas are scary. 70% of your clientele will be women, and women are almost always very intimidated by anything that's not a class. Rightfully so, because it can be intimidating going into a gym and trying new exercises for the first time. That's where you come in. The next time you go to the gym, I want you to glance into the class that's going on. What percentage of the participants are female?

Other people who you need to impress are the membership advisors and front desk. They're constantly selling packages and getting asked about training; your name needs to be at the top of their head when training inquiries are made. Buy Becky coffee at the front desk. If you hear Ted from membership likes movies, get him a gift card. Train them all. Learn about the things they like. When they refer you an assessment or client, PAY THEM IN CASH! Take 5–10% off the top and give it to them. I guarantee you if Amber in childcare or

Bill the masseuse were to get $150 bucks for a referral, they'll start talking about your services more than any other trainer. THINK OUTSIDE OF THE BOX.

Become the mayor of the gym. Smile at everyone and become that person who everyone is talking about. I never understand it when I see a trainer with their arms crossed and not smiling. As a personal trainer, you can help people live longer lives, increase their confidence, build amazing bodies, and have bootstrapping sexcapades—you're literally a life saver! Carry yourself with a positive mindset and aim at helping one person at a time. Every member needs to know who you are. Kiss babies and pet dogs; become the mayor of your gym.

Interesting

What's different between you and the other 30 trainers at your gym? How are you going to stick out? Is it your cool Koi tattoo? Or maybe you're super-hot? What if you don't have a cool tattoo or are good looking? Are you screwed? Not at all, you just need to improvise.

When I moved to the SF Bay Area from Chico, I noticed most dudes were chubby with weird-ass mustaches, and scrubby hair. I decided to get the most ripped of my life by getting down to 175lbs from 191lbs. I kept my hair clean cut like a Backstreet Boy. I didn't like being small, but I knew I would stick out. Fast forward to today; I'm hovering around 210lbs with my hair hanging halfway down my back. I was recently described by a trainer at Equinox in an email CC'd to ten other trainers as, "The big, long haired, Texas wearing everything guy walking around Equinox." People have said I could be Chris Hemsworth's body double from the movie Thor. You think I accidently came across this "new style," or was it strategy to get noticed? Being described as "the big, long-haired, Texas wearing everything guy" or "Thor's body double" gets you noticed. Getting noticed means that when people think about who they want as their trainer, they think of me.

The first thing I'd suggest in a new gym is go to the trainer's bio wall and STUDY THE LIST (most gyms have an area where they'll hang up biographies of trainers). Literally take photos of every bio and go home to analyze. You need to stand out, but be professional (don't look like a homeless person). If no one wears a hat, wear a hat. If most of the dudes are huge meatheads, get ripped. A lot of female trainers stick to body weight exercises and functional movements, so if you're a female trainer, you should learn the powerlifts. Does anyone wear glasses? If not, wear glasses. The last thing you want to do is be another sheep. Stand out!

If you haven't realized by now, the average trainer isn't very smart, and when it comes to understanding the science of personal training, there's a huge gap. That's why another way to stand out is to simply be knowledgeable. Enroll in school to master anatomy, nutrition, movement, and injuries. Take classes. Read books. Hell, sign up for the **Show Up Fitness Training Academy!** When I have a conversation with a potential client, I science all over the place. People respect individuals who know what they're talking about, so when I meet a new client, I don't show off the newest machine or flashiest exercise, I educate them on why they haven't achieved their goals. I teach them proper movements, and then overload the movements (Overload Principal 101). It seems to me that trainers today try to impress their clients by showing them "flashy" exercises. People seem to believe that new equals results. I hear all the time that "people are bored with exercise." I call BULLSHIT! Our society is tired of being fed gimmicks and not getting results. I say to my clients, "Do you want to have fun, or do you want to look amazing naked? I guarantee that if you Show Up regularly, you'll begin to have fun because you look and feel amazing. The choice is yours—Show Up, or Shut up."

This leads me into one of the most important characteristics of a trainer…

"Concocky"

There's a fine line between cocky and confident. It's a U-shaped curve. On one side, you have someone who's overly confident (cocky), which isn't sexy, it's just obnoxious or annoying. On the other, you have someone who's too passive and shy, which is equally unattractive, because they're off-putting, like they don't want to be bothered. The perfect recipe is someone in between confident and cocky, so let me introduce you to a word I thought I created (but apparently is in the Urban Dictionary), "CONCOCKY." Unfortunately in the training world, we have too many cocky trainers who abuse their power. People believe that if you're in amazing shape, you know what you're talking about. Or even scarier, people think that if you're a trainer at a gym, you're the expert. With the average trainer being cocky and in decent shape, they think they can transform anyone. This couldn't be further from the truth. Especially with the access to social media where people flaunt their bodies and sell programs that claim to yield similar results. It would be like Stephen Curry posting a workout, saying you'd soon be able to play like him if you followed his program. Does that make sense? No way! It's more complicated than that. The difference between most trainers and the ones who go through a school like **Show Up Fitness Academy** is this: The average personal trainer understands how their body works, whereas trainers who go through the **Show Up Fitness Academy** understand how the human body works and moves. The seed for confidence is planted by going to school, and your tree of knowledge will grow into a Sequoya by gaining experience and continuing your education.

Remember in *The Matrix* when Neo stopped bullets? This was the moment when he knew he was the One. There will be a point in your training career when you'll be able to stop bullets. I tell trainers that this moment will be when you 1) Fire a client, and/or 2) Receive a gift. There's nothing more empowering than knowing you have a list of people waiting to train with you. At this point in time, you'll be able to go through your clientele and fire the ones who make your life miserable. The client who bitches and complains or is always late; FIRE THEM! Obviously, do it in a professional manner,

"Mr. Jones, I'm going to have to pass you along to one of my friends who'll be able to continue to train you. The time slot of which you train at is my most popular slot and you continually show up late and aren't putting in 100% effort. As we previously discussed, I want to help you attain your goals, but I can only do so much. I wish you the best."

The other moment that helps instill confidence is when a client brings you a gift. It's very humbling when a client who's paying $60+ per hour (sometimes $200+) takes the time out of their life to get you a gift—it's an amazing feeling!

I'm like one of Pavlov's Dogs when a client walks into a training session with a brown paper bag…I know it's going to be a whiskey drinking night!

Knowledgeable/Experience

A great trainer understands anatomy, physiology, biochemistry, and bioenergetics, but can break it down into layman's terms for his or her clients. Yes, it's important to understand what the SITS muscles are and how they stabilize the gleno-humeral joint, but your client only cares about looking good naked—unless they have shoulder pain. There's no need to overwhelm them with scientific jargon. Do you think my first client was sold on the fact that I talked about the Krebs cycle (complex aerobic process in which mitochondria generate energy)? No way, it bored her to death and that's probably why she didn't sign up. I should have asked better open-ended questions, and focused more on her talking about her goals.

Talk to me once you've trained the majority of the following: obese, Type II diabetic, injured shoulder, wants to increase their Bench Press, lose fat, grow their booty, thoracic outlet syndrome, asthma, Type I diabetic, four weeks post-rhabdomyolysis, lose 20lbs in two months for a wedding, has had a heart attack, had cancer, hypothyroidism, arthritis, broken foot, herniated L5/S1, sciatica, doubled someone's squat, lateral epicondylitis, annoying, medial tibial stress syndrome, outspoken, 12 weeks out from a prep, autistic, reverse dieting, anterior knee pain, frozen shoulder, lateral knee pain, a client tells you she cheated on her husband whom you also train, torn meniscus, trained a client for three months and they gained weight (but they wanted to lose weight), six-year-old, medial knee pain, collapsed lung, DOMS to the point where they couldn't train with you for five days, pregnancy, smells (bad breath or BO), varicose veins, 90-year-old, a client who wants to train five times a week, a know-it-all, a client who doesn't want to change their diet, deaf, amputee, a client who constantly comes in hungover, farts all the time, quiet and reserved, drinks a bottle of wine a night and won't change that, had a client pass out, turf toe, trained someone who doesn't believe in weight lifting, osteoporosis, and Downs Syndrome.

I've trained every scenario above. Think of training like the game Monopoly. The goal is to get as many hotels as possible, but you must purchase one property first. Start small by training friends and family, and then progress into more challenging clientele. If you were to train at a big box gym for five years, you'd train a similar clientele.

Don't be deterred by that scary 10,000-hour rule; it's just a strong suggestion. Why not buy some of those hours by hiring top trainers to train you? The more you learn from those who've already attained those 10,000 hours, the more knowledge you're going to gain. Do you really need to spend five years in a commercial gym? Why not bust your ass and seek out the best trainers and learn from them? Don't be tightfisted with your money here. The respect that you'll get from paying others will yield dividends. If you're at a gym, pay the top trainers cash under the table—management doesn't need to know. Make sure to get a variety of training, and don't just train with one person. Think of it like college, I want you to take as many classes as possible. The more experienced and well-rounded that you become, the better you'll be. One of my trainers at Show Up Fitness gets trained at the Mecca in Venice every Friday night by a bodybuilder. He talks about his experiences and learns from the guy who's spent over 30 years under the bar. If you're new, you need to learn from as many people as you can. Start with the people in this book. From there, continue to branch out and train, read, and get those reps in. Don't be a hypocritical trainer by telling others they need a trainer, but you don't even have one yourself. You must believe in your product; hire a trainer to gain experience.

Here's Your Checklist to Be a Successful Personal Trainer:

Show Up! That means Show Up on time with a smile, work hard, and maintain a positive mindset. The average personal trainer makes between 28– and 34k their first year and quits within the first two years. Your first thought may be, "That's nothing! I can't live on 2– to 3k a month!" This, of course, depends on your circumstances. I had an 18-year-old student smile ear-to-ear when he heard that number. Two grand a month might be fine for someone right out of high school, but if you have financial obligations like a mortgage payment, a car payment, cell phone bill, children, and other expenses, and you're about to switch careers and become a personal trainer, you might be facing a harsh reality. Establishing yourself as a trainer takes time. It'll take between 6 and 12 months before you start making 2k–3k a month, and for some, it may take longer. How quickly you get there depends on your work ethic and desire. It's like the military; you can't expect to become a General within a year or two of service. Work hard, help people, continue to learn, be resilient, wake up early, be positive, and you'll do just fine as a trainer.

Build career capital. Most of you will need to spend between two and five years in a commercial gym. Train as much as possible, intern at a physical therapy clinic, and/or volunteer at a senior citizen home, at-risk youth, probation, disability home, or rehab center. The greater the variety in your experience, the better you'll become. In Cal Newport's book, *So Good They Can't Ignore You*, he discusses a term called *career capital*. Career capital is the experience you obtain over the years developing your skills. In my opinion, a lot of new trainers fail because they're impatient. In the book *Outliers* by Malcom Gladwell, he states that 10,000 is the number of hours it takes to achieve greatness. If you were to train 30 hours a week, for 52 weeks, that's 1,560 hours. It would take someone 6–7 years to obtain those 10,000 hours. For me, it took over eight years. I trained at different gyms, taught over 700 trainers, wrote over 100 blogs and articles, and now I'm finally getting some training. Does this mean I've reached my potential? No. It means I've established the required career capital to take the next step toward greatness. Show Up Fitness will soon become a household name; it just takes time. I continue to wake up early, learn, help as many people as I can, and grow with a positive mindset.

No more fluff. A good rule of thumb, if it wasn't around 40 years ago, it probably doesn't work. Corrective exercises, BOSU balls, and balancing acts should be saved for the circus. As Dan John says, "If you had 15 minutes to work out three times a week, would you spend it foam rolling and working on correctives?" I don't think so. You'd squat, hinge, press, pull, and carry heavy shit. Stop farting around with the fluff; it doesn't work!

Invest in your clients. Stop worrying about getting more clients, work on the ones that you have. If a client invests into their fitness plan, why wouldn't you invest into them? Your clients are the best form of advertising and marketing you could ever imagine, INVEST IN THEM! Each client that signs up at Show Up Fitness gets a water bottle and a shirt. If your client likes Lululemon, get them an article of clothing if they reach a milestone in their fitness journey.

Communicate clearly. Confirm client assessments and appointments. Make sure to go over the cancelation policy in detail. Don't tell your clients they're going to get into amazing shape within a few months; go over realistic expectations.

Keep yourself sane by doing things you love. Go to movies, paint, do stand-up comedy, and go on hikes. In order to avoid a burnout, you need to do things you love outside of work.

Practice what you preach. WORK OUT and be above average in a few of the following: bench, squat, deadlift, chin-ups, kettlebells, sprints, cardio, Olympic lifts, jumps, and overall physique.

Woo people with your mind, not your abs or ass. If you want to be like most narcissistic trainers today, take selfies and only highlight your body. I'll give you five years before you're begging for money on the corner. Educating people will help propel you to the top.

Be humble and kind. If you want to be successful, you need to remember why you choose this industry—to help people. Nothing is more humbling than to hear Bret Contreras talk about the glutes, or Tony Gentilcore speak on how the shoulder works.

Learn to play the game. Potential clients will judge you based off how sore they get, how many new exercises you show them, and how much they sweat. These three factors do not indicate a great workout, but you need to play the game by knowing a ton of ab, glute, and arm exercises because your clients think new exercises yield results. Slow down a few of the movements eccentrically (the negatives), which will help them FEEL THE BURN and likely cause delayed onset muscle soreness (DOMS). At the end of the workout, do a circuit so they sweat a lot. I'm all about education, but I cannot reverse all the shit a client has read or seen on social media in an hour. It's just part of the gig.

Educate your clients.

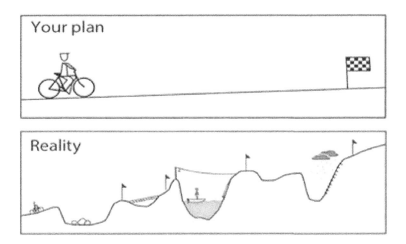

We're inundated with social media transformations and quick fixes via the media; I can only empathize. I sit every client down, show him or her this picture, and explain that change WILL take place, but it'll take time. Imagine the transformation process like 12 laps around a track (three miles). You'll finish the race, but it takes 12 laps of effort. If one lap isn't as fast as another, don't give up, adjust your speed for the laps to follow. We need to take this same approach to our New Year's Resolutions; 12 laps = 12 months. By the end of the year, you will be in a better position than you started, just like this image.

Continue your education. After you attend a 300–500-hour school like the **Show Up Fitness Personal Training Academy**, continue learning. If you want to hone in on your nutrition skills, learn via Precision Nutrition and go to ISSN nutritional conferences. Take a TRX class. Go to Perform Better workshops. Read books monthly. Your thirst for knowledge should be unquenchable.

Failure is not an option. Adopt a positive mindset and become resilient to failure. There are only two options in life, you either win, or learn; failure is for those who quit.

Learn to be uncomfortable. If you live in your comfort zone, you will have regrets. Growth comes from learning when you're knocked down. You will not get everyone to sign up and that's ok. People will say no because they don't have enough money, time, or their significant other says no. There'll be a lot of people who don't sign up with you because you lack confidence and conviction. You will have so many potential clients say no to your training services, you need to get excited about this...LEARN FROM THE EXPERIENCE. Ask them the difficult questions, "I understand that you do not want to train, and respect that. As a learning trainer, I'd love for you to give me some feedback on how I could better present training for future clients?" I know you don't want to hear it, but that's how you'll grow. If that makes you uncomfortable, send out an email and get clients' feedback. Another method is to record your assessments, and then have another trainer analyze it. Hide your phone under your desk and record the conversation. That's one hell of a learning experience.

The more you put yourself into uncomfortable positions, the better trainer you'll become. Find other ways to get uncomfortable, e.g. enroll in Toast

Masters, give talks to small groups, and take every class imaginable. (Yes, that includes, Barre, Yoga, and Pole Dancing.)

Have great hygiene. There's nothing worse than a stinker! Shower, shave, carry gum, and Axe body spray (only because the commercials are awesome).

When in doubt, refer out. If a client has red flags per the ACSM CAD Risk Stratifications, you need to refer them to a doctor before training. Unfortunately, trainers have killed people by inappropriately pushing them beyond what they're capable of. A blood pressure of 140/90 without a recent physical should first get checked out. That client could be a ticking time bomb and the last thing I want on my resume is killing a client. "My name is Chris Hitchko and I've trained 1,792 people. I've only killed one person; how would you like to train with me?" I don't think that's a bullet point I'd want on my resume.

Be creative. I once had a student who put out a Craigslist Ad that said he was leaving town and had three more sessions with a personal trainer. If someone wanted it, they needed to contact him and the sessions would be free. There was no personal trainer; it was my student luring people in with free sessions. My student was able to get three clients from this creative act. Granted, he had to train eight other people for free (and they were WEIRD), but his positive and creative mindset landed him three clients that he wouldn't have had the opportunity to train otherwise.

GET FIRED UP AND BRING ENERGY! Your clients are working 40+ hours, have shitty bosses and mean coworkers, are lonely, and have a lot of baggage. Every time they show up, you need to be 10 times more amped up then they are. Pay close attention to detail. Remember your clients' names, but the most important thing you can do is to be their Rock Star. I challenge my trainers by asking, "Would your client leave you a 5-star Yelp review today?" That answer should always be YES! Go the extra 10% and make your client experience amazing! Drink your coffee, tea, Frappuccino, WHATEVER! If you bring the energy, they will continue to SHOW UP!

Be organized. Most trainers that I come across are very unorganized. To be successful, you need to plan for the week and months ahead. Look at your calendar every Sunday night, send out your reminder texts to clients, prep food for the week, catch up on your Netflix, and plan your workouts.

Set aside 10% of paychecks for future investments and taxes. If you're working at a gym, you should put away 10% of your monthly paycheck into a savings account. $200 a month over five years will be around 15k in savings. If you started contributing $300–$500 in the last few years, you could have over 20k in savings, more than enough to start your own personal training studio. If you're an independent personal trainer, it's wise to set aside 10% from each client package that they purchase for taxes. Most trainers suck at finance. You don't want to be training at the age of 75 without any retirement, do you?

LIFE OF A TRAINER & CAREER OPTIONS

Life of a Trainer

Here's a day in the life of one of my trainers at Show Up Fitness Santa Monica.

Wake up at 4 a.m. (I challenge my trainers to wake up 2 hours before their first session to write programs, read, get their mind right, and focus on being significant.)

6 a.m. –9 a.m. Three 1-hour sessions back-to-back-to-back.

10 a.m. Eat.

11 a.m.–2 p.m. Floor shifts (We use Classpass for 1-1 training. The job of the trainer is to train and WOW the client, so they'll want to schedule a complimentary 1-1 assessment. During this 60-minute session, the trainer will discuss their goals, and try to convert them into a client. These hours are like a big box gym where you'll be given "X" amount of floor hours to "prospect" aka walk around smiling, introducing yourself to every member, and try to get assessments.

2 p.m.–5 p.m. Workout /eat.

5 p.m. –8 p.m. Train back-to-back-back.

Repeat 4–7 days a week.

Some days will be easier than others. Fridays and Saturdays are usually not as hectic—maybe half days. It's important to understand that personal trainers take the unwritten oath of training when our clients are not working; 4 a.m.–8 a.m. & 4 p.m.–8 p.m. Get used to waking up early, and going to bed late. How you handle this transition is what'll make you a successful personal trainer. I challenge students to wake up between 4–5 a.m. every day for a month. After a month of waking up at those times, you'll reprogram your brain and body to accept the morning hours. You need to constantly challenge your mindset to become successful. Are you a glass-half-full or half-empty kind of person? Learn to embrace every opportunity with a positive mindset.

Where I'd Start, If I Were Starting Now

If I were to begin my training career in 2017, I'd prefer to work at an Equinox. The facilities are premium and the structure for a personal trainer to be successful is the most complete. The average member at Equinox makes over 200k. Thus, selling your services will be easier at an Equinox compared to anywhere else. The easier the sales process becomes, the greater your confidence will grow. Confidence is key for your success. After a few years, you will have moved up the tier system (the higher tier trainer you become, the more you make), and pretty soon you can start making $50+ per session. With a proper savings plan, you could easily accumulate over 25k and within five years, and before you know it, you could own your own gym. I've had many students graduate my Academy and begin working at Equinox nationwide. I have a great relationship with their company; they are professional and focused, and there's no better place to start as a young trainer.

Then again, as I've said many times, if you Show Up, work hard, smile, and focus on helping people, you'll be successful.

How to Get Interviewed and Hired at a Corporate Gym (Equinox/Crunch/24 Hour Fitness)

Common sense states that you arrive to an interview 30 minutes early dressed appropriately, with three copies of your resume, a stellar handshake, and a personality that kills. Guess what? Common sense isn't so common anymore. Here's how to impress a hiring manager and get hired at a corporate gym.

Research the company before you go into the interview and learn about the history, expansion plans, and any sort of special certifications that they have. For example, Equinox utilizes the Functional Movement Screen (FMS) and Dr. Berardi's Precision Nutrition. Find out who's going to be interviewing you and be ready to impress them. I helped a student get a job at a Crunch in Los Angeles by looking at the hiring manager's Facebook page. We discovered that he had a huge passion for cross-country. I told the student to mention in the interview that they enjoyed cross-country. The manager then took special interest in the student and was eventually hired.

Be Prepared. You should double check the proper time and location of the interview. Review your strengths, weaknesses, and how you've handled difficult situations with clients. Why do you want to work for the company, and specifically that location? Don't be arrogant and say you have no weaknesses; they want to hear you're human. I like to be clever and state a weakness as an actual strength, "A weakness of mine is that I tend to over-commit myself to new jobs and get burned out easily. What I've learned from this is that I need to better manage my days and spend one day doing something I enjoy like fishing, hiking, or going to the movies." What did I just do? I told someone that I work too hard and I found a solution for my problem by being proactive.

Dress appropriately. Guys wear a suit; girls wear a blouse, suit, or dress pants. Don't wear fitness attire (Lululemon or Nike), and don't show off too much. Keep the girls tucked away and the dress length PG. Lastly, don't overwhelm a sensitive nose with too much cologne or perfume.

Arrive 30 minutes before the interview. Military saying goes, "If you're 10 minutes early, you're five minutes late." I don't care how much traffic there is, plan accordingly. Get there an hour early and find a coffee shop nearby. Arrive to the facility 15 minutes before the call-in time. Before you head into the interview, give yourself a pep talk by going over why you're awesome (aka braggart sheet). Testosterone levels elevate from this exercise, which in turn, increases your confidence. You are awesome—tell yourself this ten times with a smile to die for.

Bring three resumes. What if another hiring manager is present during the interview? You want to be overly prepared by having at least three resumes. Print out a one-page resume on blue or ivory colored paper that's thicker than normal. Have a few people glance over it to make sure there are no mistakes; double check punctuation, grammar, etc.

Smile and greet everyone with a firm handshake. When you meet managers and other trainers, greet them with your pearly whites and a steady handshake. Make sure it's not too hard, but not too soft or feeble. When you speak, your tone and confidence should make other candidates uncomfortable. Remember, you are the best; the job is yours.

Ask questions. I'd suggest having at least five questions to ask the interviewer. Challenge them. They want to see that you're serious about the position. Here are a few examples of good questions to ask: "What are some positive traits that you've acquired from being in the position as hiring manager?" "What are some of the fastest times that a trainer has been promoted? What characteristics did these trainers have?" "What is your policy with continuing education?" Stimulate the mind in front of you and I guarantee that they'll want you a part of the team.

Patience is a virtue. You may fit the part for the position, or you may not. Don't overwhelm management by contacting them to see how well you did or if they've decided yet. I've interviewed a lot of people and the annoying ones never made it back in.

Get business cards and network. Anyone that interviewed you, get their business card and send them a Thank You email the next day. Don't kiss ass or be needy…KISS (keep it simple, shithead.)

Hello Sarah,

Thank you for taking the time to interview me the other day. I appreciate the opportunity to be considered for the position of _____ (personal trainer at Bigfoot Spectrum). I'm looking forward to the future in the fitness industry. Have a great rest of the day.

Chris Hitchko (Tall guy with long hair / or the only girl with high heels)

Once hired, they'll provide a list of approved apparel, business cards, health insurance, retirement plans and personal training insurance (depending on the location). Health insurance should be provided after minimal training sessions are met (usually between 18 and 28 sessions per week). Some gyms may provide additional certifications and education; this is information you'd want to ask before you cross the T's and dot the I's.

Most trainers look at big box gyms negatively because the pay is minimal, i.e. it's common to get 20%–30% of a $110 per session (that's between $20 and $40/ session). This is when you start huffing and puffing until you get your way like the red-head in *Wedding Crashers*, right? Big brother is STEALING your money and you do all the work. Guess what? Life isn't fair. Instead of bitching, think about it like this. Your clients decided to train with you because of the name on the uniform, not because of you. Get over yourself. You're replaceable. Without that brand representation, you'd never be found. I challenge you to go out in the real world and get clients. In my ten-plus years of training, I've had over twenty personal trainers work for Show Up Fitness and we've trained over 300 clients. Of the 300, less than 10 were brought in from the trainers themselves. Instead, the client came because of the Show Up Fitness brand. It takes time to develop yourself as a trainer. Be excited at the opportunity to train at a big box gym and gain experience. You're getting clothes, a gym, state of the art equipment (which are expensive as hell), free advertisement, a steady check, and a brand name to represent. In five or so years, you'll be able to start your own fitness project/gym/studio.

Independent Personal Training

The life of an independent trainer isn't easy. I like to give the following example. Personal training is like fishing—you need to find fish (clients) to make a living. At a gym, you've been given a fishing rod, boots, waders, bait, and a map telling you where the best fishing is. After a few years and some hard work, you'll be one of the best fishermen around. As an independent personal trainer, it's like the beginning scene in *The Hangover* when they awoke after been roofied. You're butt-naked, without a wallet or any idea of where you are, and now it's your responsibility to find clothes, purchase equipment, and discover where the fishing poles are. It's possible to be successful, but the likelihood is slim. In my experience, most trainers fail because they do not begin their career in a gym. To be part of the small percentage who succeed, you need to have confidence, look the part, talk the part, be creative, have persistence, grit, and able to talk to anyone about why you're the best trainer. To stand out, you need client results. On top of it all, you'll need to find a place to train or buy your own gym, pay for advertisement, get business cards, develop a website, start a Yelp and Google account, and train anyone and everyone (my studio in Santa Monica is 1,000 square feet and cost 50k to start (my rent is $3,500/month). It's a grind, you got to want it more than the thousand other trainers out there. Embrace adversity because you're going to constantly be uncomfortable and thinking, am I going to make rent this month? Am I going to be able to eat? These are questions I've asked myself. Failure is not an option. Three quotes that I keep on my white board: Victory is the only option, Failing today isn't an option; fail tomorrow and Show Up or Shut Up.

A folly among trainers I see is they're either great at training, or great at business, rarely both. To succeed, you need to be a jack-of-all-trades. I wish they would've taught us in High School how to manage a business and what ROI (return on investment) or SWOT (strengths, weaknesses, opportunities, and threats) was. As a personal trainer, you need to be a great business person, but I rarely see it. If you get a check for $3,200 for 32 sessions, that $3,200 should last you four months. If you spend it all upfront on bills and toys, you're going to be working without any income for the months to come. You need to set aside 10% of each paycheck for taxes at the end of the year. If you decide to open your own gym, you should have six months of capital reserved in case of an emergency. You can pretty much write everything off, but make sure to consult with a tax advisor and read the fine print.

How Not to Burn Out

I get emails all the time from former students asking if it's normal to burnout within a few years or even months. I reply by asking what was last book they read, how many days a week are they working out, and what was the last course they took? EVERY SINGLE TIME, I never hear back from that student. Come on y'all, money doesn't grow on trees. Stop obsessing over the Instagram model and how many followers he/she has. I know you want to make a boatload of money, but it takes time, especially in the fitness industry. The most I ever made in my first five years of training was 38k. I was barely making it, and I racked up over 20k of credit card debt. To make it, you need to remember why you started this journey…YOU LOVE FITNESS AND YOU WANT TO HELP PEOPLE! If you think you're going to become Instafamous or hook up with a ton of hot chicks or dudes, stop right now; you won't make it. As with any job, you'll have your highs and lows. What separates you from the average trainer is how you adapt in this environment. To help prevent burnouts, you need to constantly be involved in things that you love. For me, I love reading, working out, watching sports, volunteering, and hanging out with my family and friends. I schedule a seminar every quarter to learn from the top minds in the industry. It never fails. Every single time, I leave those weekends motivated and FIRED UP! It's humbling to be around positive and successful coaches and trainers who've been there, done that. You'll meet great people and be reminded why you began this fitness journey; to help as many people as you can while maintaining your sanity. Training sure beats sitting behind a desk with a dickhead for a boss.

Money Matters; 75k, the Benchmark for Happiness

Studies have looked at the state of happiness and concluded that the benchmark for annual income was $75,000 a year. The lower a person's annual income falls below that amount, the unhappier they are. I'd love to be making 500k a year, but not in lieu of my health, family, relationships, or by working 80-hour workweeks and not being able to enjoy my riches. The Dalai Lama summarizes this perfectly when asked what surprises him most about humanity,

"Man surprised me most about humanity. Because he sacrifices his health in order to make money. Then he sacrifices money to recuperate his health. And then he is so anxious about the future that he does not enjoy the present; the result being that he does not live in the present or the future; he lives as if he is never going to die, and then dies having never really lived."

If you want to achieve that 75k per year happiness benchmark, here's how to do it:

75k = $6,250 per month = $3,125 per fortnightly pay check.

Let's pretend you're making $50 per session after taxes (this would be the same if you're independent or working at a gym).

$50 per session in two weeks comes down to roughly 32 sessions per week. Working 32 hours in a week doesn't sound too bad, does it? Here comes the tricky part. How many assessments does it take to get a client? How many people have you talked with to set up an assessment? I've interviewed management and directors at larger gyms and they told me that it takes around 12 points of contact to schedule an assessment. A shitty trainer will sign up 2 or 3 out of 10; top trainers will be closer to 5. (At Show Up Fitness we're around 8 out of 10.) When I hear of five clients not signing up with a trainer, I see that as five people who didn't see the value in working with you. Education and experience help those numbers increase. More opportunities will be had at a big box gym, so gain the confidence while you can, so that when you go out on your own, your closing rate will be in the 80%–90% range.

The above scenario is living in a perfect world, but what happens when a client is sick, or goes out of town on vacation? You will need to make up for these sessions and adjust your calculations. As you gain experience, you'll be able to charge more, therefore the amount of work to make 75k will become easier—but this takes time.

Supplemental Income

You can't invest all your time and energy into 1-1 training. What happens when you get sick? What happens in case of an emergency and you're out of commission for a month? God forbid, but shit happens! You need to have some working parts in place to make money while you're sleeping. What if you had ten clients, all of which bought your eBook for $9.99? That's an extra hundred bucks a month. What if you sold your clients a $20 hat, profiting by $10? What if five of those clients signed up for a $100 nutritional consultation? If you've gone through the proper schoolings (such as **Show Up Fitness Academy**), you'd be prepared to do a nutritional consultation and review food logs, images of food, calculations for BMR and protein concerns (you just can't tell clients what to eat or anything less than 1,200 calories). That would be an extra $500 a month. The point that I'm trying to make, instead of fretting over getting more clients, focus on the ones you have, and get more from them.

When Starbucks started brewing coffee, it was the world's best coffee. Through market research, they were able to determine that they could make more from the consumer by offering more. Look at what the average Starbucks has now: cake pops, sandwiches, snack packs, and doughnuts. You need to be creative on how to help your clients achieve their goals. Don't be a sales person and unload all this on them at once, it's a gradual process.

Another way to make money while you sleep is to develop quality content. It sounds easy when you jot numbers down, "I can write a book and sell it to my clients for $49," but can you even write? How do you get better at writing? WRITE MORE! You need to constantly be writing, making videos, doing vlogs, and sending out emails and texts to potential clients. Take polls on what is working, and what isn't. Use likes as a guide, but don't become too concerned with the value of a "like." As Starbucks did, listened to what the consumer wants. Whatever you try, give it a solid 30 days before you change anything. Try small group classes, cooking classes, workout groups, give talks, and go on hikes. I know a top trainer who makes over two grand a month from a book that he wrote over five years ago. That residual income must be nice, but he's also a big name. As a beginner, you need to be doing all this stuff for free, until the demand is high enough to charge a fee. Always remember this…Who are you, and what is your career capital? Unless you have a huge following, the likelihood of you making supplemental income from an eBook, blog, or YouTube page is unlikely.

You'll know when to strike while the iron is hot. If you maintain a positive mindset, SHOW UP, work hard, and listen to the words in this book, you'll be HAPPY, and making plenty of money in no time. But first, earn those stripes.

Top personal trainers in the industry weighing in on how to be successful

I interviewed some of the best trainers in the industry, top trainers of the year, and most experienced ones to compile the following list. These were the questions that I asked:

How much was your first paycheck as a trainer or if you had an internship, how long did you work without any pay?

Biggest challenge as a new trainer / something that you didn't expect?

One book every trainer should read?

If you could be a mentor to someone starting out in the industry, what would you suggest?

Most overrated aspect of the fitness industry (areas of improvement)?

Most underrated aspect of the fitness industry (biggest opportunities for growth personally / financially?)

Three people everyone should follow?

Dean Somerset – The Complete Shoulder and Hip Blueprint

1. How much was your first paycheck as a trainer or if you had an internship, how long did you work without any pay?

I think I actually owed money for having to purchase the uniform at the commercial gym. I think my second paycheck was for around a thousand dollars, which at the time was one of the biggest paychecks of my life, but was actually for a month's work, which wasn't the greatest thing going.

2. Biggest challenge as a new trainer / something that you didn't expect?

Probably understanding that you are a business now, and if you only understand the training element of things, but don't understand how to get someone in front of you or how to show them the value in your service to warrant them paying you for that service, you'll essentially be screaming into a vacuum.

3. One book every trainer should read?

The Starbucks Experience by Joseph Michelli and as a bonus read Selling the Invisible: A Field Guide to Modern Marketing by Harry Beckwith.

4. If you could be a mentor to someone starting out in the industry, what would you suggest?

Watch, observe, try, fail, re-assess, try again, find what works, improve that, find stuff you suck at, improve those, and repeat.

5. Most overrated aspect of the fitness industry (areas of improvement)?

Online training. Most people have no idea whether a program works or not, as they don't see the person doing the work, what their struggles are, or how they're actually finding success or failure. They don't understand how to coach, but want to make big bucks without working directly with people. There's nothing wrong with online training, but it's not the end-all be-all of training, and it's something I would recommend trainers against starting until they've managed to get at least 5000 in person sessions under their belt. This means at least 100 sessions a month for 4 years, and I would say it's a minimum requirement in my opinion.

6. Most underrated aspect of the fitness industry (biggest opportunities for growth personally / financially?).

Fitness experiences. People are paying a lot of money to travel for an experience, things like yoga in India, food tours in Paris, etc. so fitness tourism is a massively underserved market at the moment. There are some groups that involve elements like triathlon training in Maui to prep for the Ironman, or a spa retreat for weight loss, etc., but I would think there could be a massive opportunity for people who are regular fitness consumers who would want to have a unique experience. Maybe a trip to LA to train at Golds, have a session with a world-famous celebrity trainer, go surfing, block out Muscle Beach, etc. or something similar in New York, or a mountain retreat with hiking, mountain biking, yoga, whatever. I think people are looking to spend money on experiences, and this would be right up a lot of alleys.

7. Three people everyone should follow?

I don't know. It would depend on what they were looking to learn or get from their followers. There's a ton of options out there, and I think it's more of a matter of resonating with the individual or company. I know I turn a few people off with my style or approach, but I'm not able to make everyone happy at once, so it's not a huge concern to me. People will find the ones they want to follow through similar interests and common talk in those circles.

Bret Contreras – Ph.D. ., CSCS, "Glute Guy" and inventor of the Hip Thrust

1. How much was your first paycheck as a trainer or if you had an internship, how long did you work without any pay?

My first paycheck was for $20. I charged $20 per hour during my initial years of personal training. Laugh all you want, but my friends were making $10/hour at the time, and I was mostly training friends and family members.

2. Biggest challenge as a new trainer / something that you didn't expect?

My biggest challenge was attracting new clients. This was before the Internet was mainstream, so it wasn't as easy back then. Something I didn't expect was cancellations. If you allow them without penalty, you'll be dealing with a boatload of them so beware.

3. One book every trainer should read?

Everyone should read eMyth. It was written in the 70's I believe, but it's a quick read and it's made a huge impact on many trainer's lives.

4. If you could be a mentor to someone starting out in the industry, what would you suggest?

Don't sell out or compromise your integrity. Money is important, but your reputation is of greater importance.

5. Most overrated aspect of the fitness industry (areas of improvement)?

Supplements are the most overrated aspect of the fitness industry. Some work well, but nothing so far replaces hard work and consistency.

6. Most underrated aspect of the fitness industry (biggest opportunities for growth personally / financially?)

. Habits and behavior change and genomics represent areas of huge advancement in the industry.

7. Three people everyone should follow?

I'll give you more than three: Alan Aragon, Brad Schoenfeld, James Krieger, Eric Helms, Greg Nuckols, Chris Beardsley, Andrew Vigotsky, Spencer Nadolsky, Sohee Lee, Menno Henselmans, Stu Phillips, Layne Norton, Jeremy Loenneke, Ben Bruno, BJ Gaddour, Cem Eren, Nick Tumminello, Greg Lehman, and JB Morin.

Nick Tumminello – 2016 NSCA Personal Trainer of the Year and Owner of Performance University Fort Lauderdale, Fl

1. How much was your first paycheck as a trainer or if you had an internship, how long did you work without any pay?

My first paycheck as a personal trainer in a big-box gym – at the age of 18 – was somewhere around $500. Not very much for two-weeks pay, but I didn't have many clients to start.

2. Biggest challenge as a new trainer / something that you didn't expect?

The sale and marketing side of things. Training is a service business. The training is the service and the sales and marketing are part of business side, which is how you communicate to potential clients about what makes your service unique and valuable.

3. One book every trainer should read?

How We Know What Isn't So: The Fallibility of Human Reason in Everyday Life by Thomas Gilovich. This isn't a book about training. It's a book on how we think and how our thinking (about any subject, including training) can go wrong and lead us into holding erroneous beliefs (about training). It also discusses how we can work to think more clearly, see through conflicting information and come to better and more reliable conclusions (about training).

4. If you could be a mentor to someone starting out in the industry, what would you suggest?

Understand that most people who you'll work with as a trainer aren't going to be interested in becoming gym rats who organize their entire lives around kitchens, gyms and bathrooms.

Instead, most folks just want a great workout experience that challenges them but doesn't hurt them. And they often gauge their training success by how much they've enjoyed each workout, how they feel at the end of the workout, and by the fact they've completed a certain amount of workouts per week.

This explains why so many competent fitness professionals have long-term clients who don't look that much different and don't have impressive increases in their lifting numbers than when they started working with the trainer. But these clients are far better humans than they were when they first started because they're healthier physically and mentally.

It's okay for someone to be a recreational gym-goer who is working out for general health and fitness without focusing on any specific physique or lifting performance goals. There are many obvious benefits of exercise, like fat loss and muscle building. But in addition, there are numerous well-evidenced physical and mental health benefit.

Disease prevention, preservation of bone mass, improved mood (even in those with depression), anxiety/stress reduction, improved sleep, enhanced feeling of energy and well being, the delay of what's called "all-cause mortality" and even brain growth are part of the bigger picture.

To many clients, "getting results" from exercising isn't about achieving impressive deadlift numbers or to build a wider back – those are gym-rat goals. It simply means staying active, overcoming physical challenges, and enjoying each workout. Those are respectable goals – goals the personal trainer shouldn't look down on, but should instead encourage and be proud to help facilitate.

5. Most overrated aspect of the fitness industry (areas of improvement)?

Core training as the magic bullet of improved performance or treating back pain. I invite everyone to checkout this article I did, which discusses the research on this subject: http://shreddedbyscience.com/4-popular-beliefs-core-training-fitness-professionals-think-true/

6. Most underrated aspect of the fitness industry (biggest opportunities for growth personally / financially?)

Training seniors. Here's why:

They have very realistic goals that are more due to leading an independent lifestyle over trying to get abs.

They value the importance of regular exercise

They value professional direction because they've usually got health and injury limitations that need to be considered

They've usually got the financial stability to be regular clients.

7. Three people everyone should follow?

Bret Contreras, Brad Schoenfeld, Alan Aragon (In no particular order)

Dr. John Rusin – Doctor of Physical Therapy
1. Biggest challenges for new trainers / something they might not expect?

You must understand that to be successful for the long run in this industry, your education needs to be a continuous progress. I say "education" loosely, as I'm really referring to your self-study, mentorships, course work, certifications and even higher end level academia. They all need to continue to move forward as this will provide you an opportunity to be well versed in multiple different areas of the industry, and hopefully find your specialty niche.

2. One book every trainer should read?

Any anatomy textbook. Knowing your anatomy and what everything does from a biomechanical standpoint is a huge advantage to programming and coaching your clients. This doesn't have to be anything fancy, but it will take tons of time and energy mastering something of this magnitude. But luckily, once you have it down you'll be using this knowledge professionally for the rest of your life.

3. If you could be a mentor to someone starting out in the industry, what would you suggest?

Volunteer, get real world experience, get a mentor and ask questions. The more great coaches and trainers you can share the same air with the better. Take their knowledge and experience and apply it to your specific skill set and goals. Do that repeatedly forever.

4. Most overrated aspect of the fitness industry (areas of improvement)?

Ah there's a ton of stuff here, but I'm a big believer that you can forge your own path. Being stuck in a mill or cookie cutter approach to make money isn't for the real go-getters who want to make an impact, but it is for others. We don't just get paid to work out ourselves.

5. Most underrated aspect of the fitness industry (biggest opportunities for growth personally / financially?)

We really have a huge positive impact on the people we work with. And we get to develop strong and meaningful relationships with these people as we are the single most "in-contact" allied healthcare professional in the entire medical and fitness industry. You have an opportunity to change someone's life every single session, keep that in mind and you'll be successful.

6. Three people everyone should follow?

Christian Thibaudeau, Eric Cressey, me ;)

Dan John – Strength Coach, author, Personal Training Legend

1. Biggest challenge as a new trainer / something that you didn't expect?

Lack of a tool kit. Training muscles over movements (chest over a press). Most trainers don't know what the hell their doing. Learn the business and accounting.

2. One book every trainer should read?

Can You Go by Me, Paleo Workouts by Patrick Flynn, Death by Food – Denise Minger

3. If you could be a mentor to someone starting out in the industry, what would you suggest?

Learn more about recovery. Make it simple and get smarter on the tradition. Get an education. Have a tool kit and learn movement i.e. kettlebells/RKC, and compete in an Olympic lift.

4. Most overrated aspect of the fitness industry (areas of improvement)?

Cardio training is nonsense.

5. Most underrated aspect of the fitness industry (biggest opportunities for growth personally / financially?

Sleep, water, SHOWING UP.

6. Three people everyone should follow?

Bret Contreras, B.J. Fogg, Josh Hillis / Percy Cerutty

Charles Staley – Coach, author, Personal Training Legend

1. How much was your first paycheck as a trainer or if you had an internship, how long did you work without any pay?

I put this question down because social media seems to glorify personal training into a profession that pays millions without working hard- so far from the truth. My first paycheck was less than a grand.)

So, in my previous life I was a martial arts instructor (which is a quasi-fitness-related career I suppose), and then right after that, I got a job running the weight room at a YMCA in Poughkeepsie New York. And honestly, I don't recall what I made at that job, but it was enough to get by as a guy in his 20's.

One point I should make is that I've never been a trainer exclusively. Ever since my start in the fitness industry, I've done a combination of training, teaching, writing, consulting, etc. This is because I've got various skills and interests, but strategically, it's also a way to make sure you don't have all your eggs in the same basket so to speak. Always seek to have multiple streams of income.

2. Biggest challenge as a new trainer / something that you didn't expect?

Well, I'm trying to think back on being a new trainer (which I was in the late '80's lol)... for me I think it was just the fact that the idea of personal training was not familiar to most people at the time — the word had been coined, but most people weren't really familiar with the concept. But aside from that, one annoying thing for me was simply clients who had their own idea of what they should be doing, and who got annoyed if you didn't play along. In other words, people who pay for your expertise, but who aren't willing to do what you want them to do. Much later in my career, it because clearer to me that you have to meet people where they live so to speak — there are certain expectations they have, and certain things you have on your agenda for them. When you train people, it can't be a dictatorship — you have to give people a little of what they want, even if you disagree — this builds trust, and then later, you can impose you will on them ;-)

3. One book every trainer should read?

I REALLY like Greg Nuckol's *Art And Science Of Lifting* book set (2 volumes). It's a fantastic resource for people looking to get a clear understanding of the scientific underpinnings of training in a way that's easy to comprehend.

4. If you could be a mentor to someone starting out in the industry, what would you suggest?

Oh there is so much, I guess holistically, it's important to do some self-analysis about whether you really want to make a <u>business</u> of training people, or whether it's more of just a temporary thing or a hobby for you. If it's the former, you need to become really astute about marketing, branding, money management, personal productivity, sales, and so on. Now I'm not suggesting that you ignore your fitness education and just be a shitty trainer, but when you look around, the most financially successful trainers tend to not be the best trainers per se, they just understand business. If you find that off-putting, you might reconsider being a professional trainer.

5. Most overrated aspect of the fitness industry (areas of improvement)?

So there is a category of philosophies/activities/methods that might be loosely termed "corrective exercise" (and/or core stability, and/or posture training), and this movement seems to be turning every personal trainer into a wannabe Physical Therapist. Suddenly (well, this has been percolating over the past 20 years to be more accurate) everyone is dysfunctional and in need of all sorts of exotic exercises involving physio balls, bands, Bosu Balls, foam rollers, manual resistance/assistance, and so on.

The funny thing is, if you go back maybe 30 years or so, no one seemed to have all these problems! Up until that time, people just lifted weights, and funny enough, they got really big and strong. But today, everyone is a physical therapy patient without a Physical Therapist.

I saw a young guy in the gym just yesterday actually, probably 6'3", 180 pounds, really skinny, and for over 45 minutes I watched him do all sorts of shoulder rehab drills with bands, foam rolling, and so on. Don't get me wrong, stuff like that can have a place, but that's all he did. And while this is anecdotal, while he was doing all of that, I'm on the other side of the room at age 57 deadlifting 385 for sets of 10. I never stretch, never activate my core or awaken my glutes, never do correctives, I just do basic lifts and I have no injuries, no pain anywhere, despite lifting 4-5 times a week for almost 35 years now.

So I guess what I'm saying is that a lot of people tend to get ahead of themselves and lose perspective sometimes. Yes, if you have a compelling reason to think that you have an injury or gluteal amnesia or whatever, get that shit fixes. But if you're going to use "correctives," do so strategically, not reflexively. Have a reason for everything you do.

6. Most underrated aspect of the fitness industry (biggest opportunities for growth personally / financially?)

To this I've gotta say, I believe in the idea of "if you build it, they will come." Meaning, whatever you're truly passionate about, there are others who are too, and these people need a leader. Here's an example: if 30years ago, if I gathered my gym buddies together and said "OK, so I have an amazing idea: I'm going to combine powerlifting, gymnastics, weightlifting, distance running, kettlebell lifting, and a bunch of other stuff together into one workout, and to top it off, I'm going to make a central website where I post a new workout every day, and it'll be TOTALLY random too — like a workout might be something like snatching 135 for as many reps as possible in 3 minutes, followed by muscle ups, then 100 burpees, and finally a 3 mile run," people would think I'd lost my mind. But today, the guy who thought of that is a very wealthy man. And he's not the only one, nor is Crossfit the most unlikely example — check out something called "Functional Patterns": it's kind of like L. Ron Hubbard had a mushroom trip at a gym, I kid you not. Your idea is too crazy you say? Mmm, probably not.

So my advice is, cultivate your passions, share them with the World, and remember, you don't need everyone to join your tribe

7. Three people everyone should follow?
Eric Helms, Greg Nuckols, and Alan Aragon.

Kellie Hart (Davies) – Owner at Fit Philosophies & Co-Author of Strong Curves.

1. How much was your first paycheck as a trainer or if you had an internship, how long did you work without any pay?

I might not be the best resource as my career is rather unconventional. I wrote Strong Curves with Bret before I became a trainer. While finishing the book, I took a brief job at a local gym and hated it. So I bought my own equipment and started training clients at my house.

2. Biggest challenge as a new trainer / something that you didn't expect?

The time constraints. Depending on your gym setting, you aren't given ample time to work with clients. It was one of the largest reasons I purchased my own gym equipment. I didn't like the turn-and-burn atmosphere of the commercial gym.

3. One book every trainer should read?

Strong Curves, of course. I honestly feel that trainers get tons of continued education, but don't learn enough about business. All the fitness knowledge in the world won't make you a good business person, and in the end you won't be happy.

So I recommend getting a solid business education. How to manage personal finances, clientele, market and build your own brand. You may start out working in a facility, but you don't want to sell for that company forever. If you are good at what you do you will eventually want to branch out on your own.

A book that transfers well to all aspects of your career is *7 Habits of Highly Effective People*. *As A Man Thinketh* by James Allen is another great one.

4. If you could be a mentor to someone starting out in the industry, what would you suggest?

Find your niche by honing in on your passion early on. Don't try to bend to what you think the market wants. Be true to yourself always, be authentic as hell, and deliver above and beyond anyone's expectations. That will always work in your favor.

5. Most overrated aspect of the fitness industry (areas of improvement)?

Marketing hype is always an area of contention for those of us who are truly passionate about helping people. Fads, quick fixes, and dangerous diets, supplements and workouts loom around every corner. The best thing to do is turn off the noise and do your best work. You're not competing with fads. You are building a career for a lifetime. Fads and trends come and go, but your compassion and knowledge are timeless.

6. Most underrated aspect of the fitness industry (biggest opportunities for growth personally / financially?)

Hybrid online/in person programs. Working with clients in person is such an incredible aspect of your career, but you are always trading time for dollars. And when a client cancels, you lose money.

Building hybrid programs that service clients both on and off-line help you generate income while you sleep.

7. Three people everyone should follow?

Dr. Zachary Long, Dr. John Rusin, Dean Somerset

Tony Gentilcore – Master Jedi Knight, Co-founder of Cressey Performance, blogger, and Personal Trainer (www.tonygentilcore.com)

1- How much was your first pay check as a trainer or if you had an internship, how long did you work for without any pay?

After I did my student teaching my senior year in college (I was going to be a health teacher, but soon realized that 1) wearing a tie every day sucked balls and 2) teaching middle schoolers sex education wasn't the most fun thing in the world to do. Luckily, I also had to complete an internship for my concentration (in Health/Wellness Promotion), and ended up landing a sweet gig at a corporate fitness center just outside of Syracuse, NY. It lasted the entire summer and the only payment I received was a handshake and a job afterwards. The stars aligned and it just so happened the place where I was interning had opened up another full-time position by the time my internship was over, which meant I was able to wear sweatpants to work everyday. Score! If I remember correctly that job netted me around 20K for the year. Granted it was middle-of-no-where central NY, so the cost of living was pretty low, but my average paycheck was $380 per week. Lets just say I wasn't buying grass-fed beef back then.

2-   Biggest challenge as a new trainer / something that you didn't expect?

Honestly, the nuances of being a "people person." School doesn't prepare you for when a real, live, in-the-flesh, person is standing there in front of you and you have to, you know, have a conversation with them. Some of my first training sessions were pretty freakin awkward. Lots of weird, awkward silences or me quoting Lord of the Rings. "You shall.....not......PASS!!!!' Being a good training isn't all about knowing the nuts and bolts of assessment, program design, and exercise technique. It helps, for sure, but it's not the "x-factor." The x-factor is not being an asshole. Not being an asshole = avoid being the pretentious know-it-all who tries to talk over people's heads and win them over with big words like synergistic dominance, reciprocal inhibition, feed forward loops, or apical expansion. Most clients could care less and probably think you're tool if you speak to them that way. Not being an asshole = being a people person. Being able to talk about movies, television shows, music, their kids, their partner, their dog, the shitty LA traffic. Not being an asshole, and learning people skills is a vast challenge for many new trainers.

3-   One book every trainer should read?

I'm going to cheat and say this: I think the best trainers, and those who do really well are avid readers and diverse readers. Meaning, they don't only read training and nutrition books.

Don't get me wrong: it's important to read books related to our field in order to get better, but I also encourage new trainers to expand their literary portfolio and read other books too: fiction, non-fiction, business/personal development, Kama Sutra, etc if for no other reason to be well-rounded human being.

Training: I don't necessarily agree with all he says in the book (particularly with regards to some of his squatting cues) but Starting Strength by Mark Rippetoe is an excellent book every incoming trainer should read.

***I will say, too, that books can become outdated pretty quickly. This is why it's important to stay in tune with the popular fitness blogs so you know what some of the fitness super stars area thinking TODAY. Too, I'd HIGHLY recommend subscribing to research reviews. My "go to's" are:

- MASS - Monthly Applications in Strength Sport

- Alan Aragon Research Review

- Strength & Conditioning Research Review (Bret Contreras)

- Business: Give and Take by Adam Grant. Cliff Notes: those who tend to be the most successful in any field are those who pay it forward.

4-   If you could be a mentor to someone starting out in the industry, what would you suggest?

Well, I've been told by others I am a mentor to them, so that's cool. I guess the one thing I'd suggest is don't be an uppity douche and charge people to come shadow you or observe. I've written on this on several occasions, but I never understand why some coaches do this. When I was at Cressey Sports Performance we always had an open-door policy. Anyone who wanted to come in to watch for a day (or two) were more than welcome to do so. We had nothing to hide. I follow this same policy now that I'm on my own. Anyone who reaches out to ask to stop by or come hang out for an afternoon are more than welcome to.

5 Most overrated aspect of the fitness industry (areas of improvement)?

The idea that distance coaching is easy. It's not. Many trainers have aspirations of ditching their commercial gym gig in lieu of setting up some distance coaching empire, where they'll be able to live anywhere and travel the world......all while working with people over their laptop. Let me tell you that it's NOT that easy. This isn't to say I don't feel there's a way to make distance coaching a viable source of income for some people, but the whole idea that it's easier is BS. It can be waaaaaaaaay more time consuming than people think, and I'd recommend, highly, to try not to be seduced by all those Facebook Ads you see from trainers saying you'll make six-figures within two months if you only follow their system.

6-   Most underrated aspect of the fitness industry (biggest opportunities for growth personally / financially?)

I think it behooves any trainer to work on his or her's writing skills. It's a saturated market out there - everyone has a blog - but those who write well, write good, actionable content, and do so consistently, will always float to the top.

7-   Three people everyone should follow?

Everyone knows Dan John, Eric Cressey, Mike Robertson, Bret Contreras, blah blah blah. Here are a few AMAZING coaches you should follow: Joel Seedman, Lee Boyce, Lori Lindsey

Ben Bruno – Celebrity Trainer in Los Angeles, CA

1. How much was your first paycheck as a trainer or if you had an internship, how long did you work without any pay?

I took an unpaid internship with Mike Boyle for I think 4 months. Trainers that work for people always bitch by saying the owner / gym take the lions share. Trainers complain too much and think the gym / owner doesn't do shit. You never realize how hard is until you get out there on your own trying to find clients. I wasn't certified for a while (I had a sociology major), the internship and deliberate practice help get me to where I am today.

2. Biggest challenge as a new trainer / something that you didn't expect?

I liked sports and lifting weights, I didn't realize the long hours that came with the job- like really long, really early, really late hours. Get used to a lot of long days.

3. One book every trainer should read?

I'm not a big book reader. I think Boyle wanted us to read how to win / influence people. Outliers by Gladwel was good. People tend to get a shit ton of certs without the deliberate practice.

I'm all about interpersonal skills over the X's and O's.

4. If you could be a mentor to someone starting out in the industry, what would you suggest?

Do an internship especially with someone who you respect and something you want to do. If you're into body building / physique, a PT (physical therapy) internship isn't for you. So many facets within the fitness world, pick what you're interested in and train TONS of people for free. When I was interning at Boyles, I trained a lot of volume and everything between 10-75. Train everyone.

5. Most overrated aspect of the fitness industry (areas of improvement)?

Online training. Trainers are quick at having an end goal of getting out of training but lack the actual training. I train 7 days a week an. To be a successful internet person you have to be doing it. I'm good at what I do because I'm doing it, not talking about doing it.

6. Most underrated aspect of the fitness industry (biggest opportunities for growth personally / financially?)

Being a great communicator. I don't take new clients, because I don't lose clients. A big part of picking a trainer is choosing to be with someone for 3-4 hours. Personality is huge and a lot of trainers just talk and annoying. It's the same talk. I don't see much deliberate practice. Too many trainers are great at TALKING, but don't practice it. Work ethic and having a personality.

7. Three people everyone should follow?

Boyle – mentor, Bret Contreras, Don Saladino (New York nice smart guy)

Eric Bach – Owner of Bach Performance in Denver Colorado

1- How much was your first pay check as a trainer or if you had an internship, how long did you work for without any pay?

My first paycheck?

Absolutely zero. At one point, I was part of a community fitness program at 5:00 am until 8:00 am, then moving on to an local Sports Performance gym for six hours per day for a semester.

2- Biggest challenge as a new trainer / something that you didn't expect?

Honesty, I had no idea I needed to run a business. Sure, my skills as a trainer were solid, but I had no idea how to reach people, how to market, nor how to sell. Yes, you can be a great coach, but if you can't get people in front of you and convert them in to clients, then you're not providing the value you're capable of.

3- One book every trainer should read?

The Power of Less by Leo Baubata

Simplicity drives action. By taking the lessons in this book and applying them to your clients, you'll be able to help them stop feeling overwhelmed and take massive action.

4- If you could be a mentor to someone starting out in the industry, what would you suggest?

Focus on becoming the best trainer you can first before getting side tracked by the idea of online training, writing, creating products. You need time in the trenches.

5- Most overrated aspect of the fitness industry (areas of improvement)?

Oh wow. Where to start? I'm going to cover an overarching issue: absolutism. There's a trend to belief/ say one training method, dietary style, or activity is best. You need to count macros. You need intermittent fasting. Strength first, you need to start powerlifting. CrossFit or die. You see what I mean? All training and all diets can work. For your clients, you need to determine which methods resonate with them, are conducive to creating long-term habits, and improve their life rather than consume it. Everything can work. The only absolute in fitness is there are NO absolutes for every client.

6- Most underrated aspect of the fitness industry (biggest opportunities for growth personally / financially?)

Instead of trading dollars for hours and selling personal training packages, sell solutions. If it's going to take a client six months to lose 40 pounds, that's what you should offer.

Be up front about what it will take your clients to achieve their desired result. Not only will this set realistic expectations, but you'll get more buy in with your coaching from the start.

7- Three people everyone should follow?

John Berardi/ Precision Nutrition

Eric Cressey

Jon Goodman/ thePTDC

Tim Henriques – Director of Education Va-Md-Dc National Personal Training Institute

1. How much was your first paycheck as a trainer or if you had an internship, how long did you work without any pay?

My first PT job was actually a salaried job where I got paid the same amount and just trained clients. Kind of like being a banker but I was a trainer, worked every day 6-2. I was making 35k a year so I guess the check was like $1,350 before taxes.

2. Biggest challenge as a new trainer / something that you didn't expect?

The number of cancellations is staggering, when my gym did an analysis 20% of all scheduled sessions were canceled. For a full-time trainer that is 1-2 sessions a day that will be canceled. Have a cancelation policy that is in writing, the client agrees to it, you think it is fair, and that you are comfortable enforcing it. Many new PT's let the clients walk all over them and that establishes a terrible precedent. It is much better to start off strict then the other way around. In this day age of social media be very clear about how a client can cancel the session (and what isn't a viable option).

3. One book every trainer should read?

How much of an a-hole will I be if I say one of my books? Whatever, they are out there and I am not afraid of a shameless plug. Read their reviews on amazon and see if they are a good fit for you. If you want to be a career trainer that really understands the body read my text NPTI's Fundamentals of Fitness and Personal Training; if you just like lifting and you work with barbells (even if you don't compete) then read All About Powerlifting.

4. If you could be a mentor to someone starting out in the industry, what would you suggest?

Since my full-time job is getting people ready to become a trainer, I am thinking of a million things for this, such as get a good education (go to school, don't self-study this topic), shadow real world training, and practice on friends and family. But I think at the heart of it one needs to do this:

Be passionate about some aspect of fitness

Train yourself to a reasonably high level in that aspect of fitness – remember, you are your first client.

Train your clients in a manner that you would like to be trained (this doesn't mean only train them based on your goals, but give them workouts you would enjoy going through)

Don't make a client do something you have never done yourself

5. Most overrated aspect of the fitness industry (areas of improvement)?

The whole posture = pain and that everyone moves broken and we must do odd little exercises to fix you is annoying. It became super popular in the late 90's and early 2000's and has stuck around. Initially there was some small science to back it up, now most of that has been debunked, and yet it still sticks. Good news is those workouts get shit for results so they won't be around too

Chris Hitchko CSCS

long, thirty years from now no one will be training like that. But getting stronger and little bit more jacked will still be in style.

6. Most underrated aspect of the fitness industry (biggest opportunities for growth personally / financially?)

I may be old school but the person that simply shows up, every time, on time, ready to do their job, if they combine that with the 4 bullet points above and they have at least adequate social skills, should be able to be successful. Make the client a very high priority. I have talked to many people that had to fire their trainer because the person wasn't dependable, even though they like working with the trainer when they were there. If you cancel more than 1 out of 50 sessions with a client with minimal notice, that is a big problem.

7. Three people everyone should follow?

That is a tough one. Lots of good people out there (might be better to make a list of popular people NOT to follow) but most people are niche so if aren't into that niche their info may not be that useful to you.

Bret Contreras, Bryan Krahn, Ben Bruno

Nik Herold – Regional Educational Manager at 24-hour Fitness

1. How much was your first paycheck as a trainer or if you had an internship, how long did you work without any pay?

Around $750 at my 1st training gig at a small private studio in Anaheim

2. Biggest challenge as a new trainer / something that you didn't expect?

It's a toss up between sales and prospecting and writing a good program -- not workouts -- for clients. But remember you can't write a program if you don't have a client. Learn how to sell and work on that every single day for twice as long as you work on other stuff until you become great at it.

3. One book every trainer should read?

Switch by Chip and Dan Heath

4. If you could be a mentor to someone starting out in the industry, what would you suggest?

Get a coach for your business and program design. If you can't afford a coach, volunteer or do an internship. Take them out for coffee weekly -- just find a way to get great coaching. The best coaches have coaches and you'll want to model after people with success. Learn from their successes and failures.

5. Most overrated aspect of the fitness industry (areas of improvement)?

The most overrated aspect is that new always equals better. That goes for equipment and the "enter-training" exercises you see on YouTube and Instagram. There's a reason barbells and squats have been around forever -- they still get great results.

6. Most underrated aspect of the fitness industry (biggest opportunities for growth personally / financially?)

The biggest area for growth is not sets and reps, but COACHING. You can know all the science, but if you don't know how to coach different types of people they'll never do your program

7. Three people everyone should follow?

Dr. John Berardi, Paul Chek, Mark Verstegem, Bonus person – Thomas Plummer

Magen Mintchev – Personal Trainer & Reebok One Ambassador, Houston, Tx

1. How much was your first paycheck as a trainer or if you had an internship, how long did you work without any pay?

At a big box gym, it was peanuts! I immediately wondered if I made the right decision to move from corporate to training. Six months into that first gig, I relocated to a boutique gym. MUCH happier and much better pay!

2. Biggest challenge as a new trainer / something that you didn't expect.

For me, at the first gym I was at, was having to push their products. I didn't like the products and I didn't believe in them so it was hard for me to sell them. I didn't feel right selling them to my clients.

3. One book every trainer should read?

How about two? "The Vulgar Truth Diet: Fat Loss" by Chris Hitchko and "Ignite the Fire" by Jon Goodman

4. If you could be a mentor to someone starting out in the industry, what would you suggest?

Market yourself and do it well. Find your niche. Be consistent. Start a blog, utilize social media, run campaigns, get sponsored (by companies you believe in), build relationships, use your resources, network.

5. Most overrated aspect of the fitness industry (areas of improvement)?

Instagram trainers who aren't even certified! They have a huge following because of their looks (nothing bad about that), but they decide to take advantage of their followers and put out workouts and meal plans without being certified. STOP DOING THIS. And…STOP BUYING INTO THIS!

6. Most underrated aspect of the fitness industry (biggest opportunities for growth personally / financially?)

Online / Skype workouts. It can be done and it should! Online is where everything is headed–figure out a way to train people from the comfort of your own home or your own gym (if you have one you own).

7. Three people everyone should follow?

Bret Contreras, Nick Tumminello, Girls Gone Strong

Andy Haley - CSCS, Performance Director STACK.COM

1. How much was your first paycheck as a trainer or if you had an internship, how long did you work without any pay?

I have a bit of a unique situation being on the media side of the fitness industry. For better or worse, I focused most of my time in college in labs rather than on the training floor. I was planning to go to PT or Chiropractic school, but got a job at STACK a few months after I graduated. So, I was fortunate to immediately have a salaried job right out of school.

2. Biggest challenge as a new trainer / something that you didn't expect?

The biggest challenge for me was information overload. So many great trainers and coaches publish amazing content online, and a lot of that content came directly through me in my position at STACK. At first I tried to incorporate every single great philosophy, methodology or exercises into my programming.

When I look back at my early programs, it's a total face palm moment. The workouts were a bit of a cluster f*$# because I was trying to include too much.

Over the years I've developed my own programming philosophy inspired by several mentors. That said, I still take great ideas from other coaches apply them where it makes sense. However, they are tools in my toolbox rather than mandatory additions to my workouts.

The KISS (Keep it Simple Stupid) principle is truly the way to go.

3. One book every trainer should read?

Functional Training for Sports by Michael Boyle

4. If you could be a mentor to someone starting out in the industry, what would you suggest?

Don't be clever just for the sake of being clever with your exercises and programming. Everything should have a purpose. If you can't explain why you're having someone do a movement, chances are it shouldn't be in your workouts.

5. Most overrated aspect of the fitness industry (areas of improvement)?

Top certifications should be reserved for those with formal education or proven experience. It's frustrating to hear about people who one day decide to become a personal trainer or strength coach and are able to get a 'reputable' certification with no background in the industry. It devalues the certification process and the profession as a whole.

6. Most underrated aspect of the fitness industry (biggest opportunities for growth personally / financially?)

I'd have to say the most underrated aspect of the fitness industry is your ability to build your brand online. I've had a few folks start contributing to STACK right out of college and their online presence and proven understanding of training concepts eventually helped them land jobs at some of the top training facilities in the country.

I think every single trainer should write online, whether that's on a personal site, STACK, T-Nation or even on forums like StrengthCoach.com. Share your knowledge, build credibility, get your name out there, educate others and start a discussion on your ideas and philosophy.

And you might be able to earn some extra cash in the process.

7. Three people everyone should follow?

Tony Gentilcore, John Rusin and Joel Seedman (and Mike Boyle, of course).

Mike Beatrice – The Movement, Oakland, CA

1. How much was your first paycheck as a trainer or if you had an internship, how long did you work without any pay?

When I first became a trainer I wanted to work for myself from day 1. I had to generate my own leads/clients through very little resources. I landed my first client who paid me a measly 30$ per session in his garage in Hayward. I used to spend more money on gas and being stuck in traffic then the job was even worth. Shortly after I started doing a bunch of gorilla type marketing with flyers and postcards and free bootcamps etc. I was able to build up a really solid PT business that was making me over 6 figures in my second year.

2. Biggest challenge as a new trainer / something that you didn't expect.

I didn't expect my already existing hospitality skills to have such a huge place in the equation for building a successful business. The best clients are long term clients whom you will build a solid relationship with. Basically you need to create a lot of regular customers. This is something the majority of trainers lack. If you see a trainer who is constantly trying to sell something I can assure you that you are looking at a trainer who is struggling to get a lot of clients. The best programs sell themselves. Biggest challenge is that the industry is watered down with so much garbage and people are window shoppers. They shop around for price and think of every trainer as being the same. How sadly mistaken people are for believing this garbage. So I guess the challenge is that a lot of other trainers are idiots and they are going around underselling quality coaching by watering down the market with Groupons and 30-day challenges.

3. One book every trainer should read?

I'm a fan of Eric Cressey and Mike Boyle. Good quality athletic based info particularly around shoulder, hip and spine focus.

4. If you could be a mentor to someone starting out in the industry, what would you suggest?

Wake up early, grind all day and be relentless until you get the results you want. Set goals and stay aggressive in your pursuit of knowledge while growing your business. Teach your clients a better habitual lifestyle and how to move properly and they will be a client for life. Client retention is your number one goal with every client that is how your business will succeed. Do not hurt your clients by doing stupid meaningless exercises that look cool and deliver negative results. Brand yourself. Be recognizable. Find a lane and don't expect to appeal to everyone. Find out who you are and be that and kill it!

5. Most overrated aspect of the fitness industry (areas of improvement)?

Personal trainers are overrated because there are so many of them and quite frankly they're a dime a dozen. Until you decide to put in the necessary effort needed to succeed you are just going through the motions of another dead-end job. Get knowledgeable. Practice your craft. Practice what you preach. Stay diligent.

30-day challenges that promise extreme weight loss. This is a lifestyle; better habits must be learned. Don't convince your clients you're the best by beating them down physically so they can lose a few pounds. Help them move better and create habits that make long term manageable weight loss obtainable. They will thank you, I promise.

Crunches and sit-ups will never give you the "abs" you want.

Fasted cardio is like a dog chasing his tail in my opinion.

Piss poor kettlebell and barbell coaching. Just put them down if you don't know how to use them properly. Or learn how to use them properly. Educate yourself to possess the skill set to properly coach movements utilizing these "popular" pieces of equipment

Juice cleanses for weight loss. Never gonna happen!!! Eat right. Eat clean. Exercise. Stay the course.

Waist trainer belts. Need I say more?

6. Most underrated aspect of the fitness industry (biggest opportunities for growth personally / financially?)

I think the most underrated aspect is movement quality control. A proper push, pull, squat, hinge and carry will make for a solid athlete. With the overabundance of high impact, high intensity interval training programming that is coveted across the world, there is not nearly enough emphasis on the quality of the actual movement. Most bodies are not prepared to perform a large majority of these exercises and movement patterns that are common in these larger group environments. More time needs to be spent on mobility, calisthenics, dynamic and static stretching as well as foam rolling. There are too many unnecessary injuries.

7. Three people everyone should follow?

Gray Cook, Kelly Starrett, Eric Cressey

Dre Dos Santos – CSCS, independent trainer Honolulu, Hawaii

1. How much was your first paycheck as a trainer or if you had an internship, how long did you work without any pay?

First check was $1300. Prior to that I was unpaid intern for about 4 months.

2. Biggest challenge as a new trainer / something that you didn't expect?

Handling different personalities and selling.

3. One book every trainer should read?

I can't pick one book. Essentialism, Mindset, The War Of Art.

4. If you could be a mentor to someone starting out in the industry, what would you suggest?

Focus on building relationships

5. Most overrated aspect of the fitness industry (areas of improvement)?

I loathe marketing tactics. Word-of-mouth referrals are gold.

6. Most underrated aspect of the fitness industry (biggest opportunities for growth personally / financially?)

People don't realize that word of mouth is the bloodline of your business.

7. Three people everyone should follow?

Jon Goodman, everybody from Cressey Sports Performance.

Robert Gomez – NPTI Graduate – Personal Trainer in SF Bay Area

1. How much was your first paycheck as a trainer or if you had an internship, how long did you work without any pay?

$438.50 (to be exact) was my first check

2. Biggest challenge as a new trainer / something that you didn't expect?

Going from selling gym memberships, to working with people a few times a week on a personal level. I found that getting someone involved without being pushy was a challenge. Also, being able to smoothly adjust to different personalities and clients (I overthought a lot in the beginning)

3. One book every trainer should read?

Ignite the Fire. Tools of Titans is a book I'm currently enjoying. The book covers interviews from some of the most successful athletes, actors and business men/women. You can bounce around the book with sections being of health, wealth, and wisdom.

4. If you could be a mentor to someone starting out in the industry, what would you suggest?

I'd suggest not overthinking, and putting your ego aside. Be a sponge for knowledge. Don't assume someone will or won't purchase training due to looks. I currently have a client who came in at 320lbs, smelled, chewed tobacco, had food in his beard and from the looks of it, wasn't going to buy any training. Nobody thought he'd commit, let alone purchased 16 sessions a month for $1120. Remember why you got into training, to help people. I gave the client an assessment, asked open ended questions, and glad to say I've been training him for over nine months.

5. Most overrated aspect of the fitness industry (areas of improvement)?

AMRAP's. You gotta max out or perform AS MANY REPS AS POSSIBLE!

6. Most underrated aspect of the fitness industry (biggest opportunities for growth personally / financially?)

Accountability. It's not just about our 60 minutes 2-3 times a week but also keeping up with their food/water intake, moving on days off, sleep, stress, etc.

7. Three people everyone should follow?

1) Bret Contreras, 2) Accelerate Sports Performance, and 3) Ben Bruno.

Chris Hitchko – Teacher, Show Up Fitness Owner, and Personal Trainer.

1. How much was your first paycheck as a trainer or if you had an internship, how long did you work without any pay?

Less than $400 at Bladium. For the first three years of my training career, I spent my life commuting between two-different training jobs- one in Alameda, CA, and the other in Walnut Creek. Seven years later, my first bi-monthly paycheck was… wait for it, this sucker is going to blow your undies off…$1,936. My gym in Santa Monica is scheduled to generate over 300k in revenue 2017 and within my first month of owning my own Personal Training Academy, I made more than I did in 6-months of teaching at my highest rate. PATIENCE IS A VIRTUE.

2. Biggest challenge as a new trainer / something that you didn't expect?

Sales and building relationships. As a new trainer, you don't know what your value is. My mindset was, "Screw you, stay unhappy and fat if you don't want to train with me." That mentality didn't work. It took me many years to understand the value of building rapport, listening, and focusing on one person at a time. Learn to ask questions with intent, not just to follow the question up with your own blabber. Asking someone how their day is, followed up by, tell me about something interesting that you've learned at your job in the past few weeks? Genuinely get to know people, not the superficial bullshit.

3. One book every trainer should read?

The Vulgar Truth Diet: Fat Loss II (when it comes out in spring of 2017.) You'll learn how to fix your S.P.I.N.E. (Stress, Sleep, Sex, Psychology, Injuries, Nutrition, and Exercise), and laugh your ass off. The name says it all, so if you can't handle vulgarity or crass drawings, you may want to skip it. It's 2017 and we're all such delicate little snowflakes, or as Elon Musk says in his book, "We've grown fucking soft" in response to people taking weekends off. Musk's & Phil Knight's *Shoe Dog* are fucking amazing.

4. If you could be a mentor to someone starting out in the industry, what would you suggest?

Don't be transactional. Most trainers push too hard for the sale and once the client says no, they forget about them. Great trainers will follow up, put them into an email list, send them bi-weekly articles, call them on their birthday to offer a free session, and truly look out for their best interest. The moment you drop the ego and focus on helping others, you'll succeed.

Read more.

Wake up early.

Turn emotional pain into physical pain - no one cares about your problems; WORKOUT!

Be open to change. Science is constantly challenging our beliefs. A great trainer will continue to learn and evolve. Imagine if we didn't evolve, we'd still be putting leeches on our bodies when we get sick. Don't be that trainer still putting leeches on your clients!

5. Most overrated aspect of the fitness industry (areas of improvement)?

NASM, the entry standards to become a personal trainer and quest for more certifications. My displease for NASM began in 2009. I was a trainer for three years with a degree in Kinesiology and ACSM certified, and told by my boss (who I later blackmailed because she was sleeping with another trainer), that I needed to get NASM certified. I told her, "You mean the BOSU ball cert?" Unless you want to work with a special population (cancer, coronary artery disease, athletes), you don't need MORE certifications. It's big brothers' way of taking more money from you. After you establish a foundation by going to school, doing an internship, and taking courses from the industries best, you don't "need" any more certifications, especially the 8+ that NASM offer- GIVE ME A BREAK! I despise NASM only trainers. Sure, some of their foundational aspects in anatomy, nutrition, and physiology are current, but a lot of it is outdated i.e. overactive and underactive muscles, adhesions, and their hypertrophy model blows. To be a successful personal trainer you need to learn anatomy, the movement patterns (which they don't even teach you), and proper overload, not pad your resume with more of their acronyms. Anytime I see a trainer with NASM-CPT, CES, PES, FNS, and/or WLS, I laugh and don't even give that "trainer" the time of day. If you are a cert whore, get one from each of the top associations and take the best information to help your clients reach their goals.

6. Most underrated aspect of the fitness industry (biggest opportunities for growth personally / financially?)

Smiling & reciprocity. I've been to so many commercial gyms; I rarely see trainers smile. The notorious RBDF (resting bitch /dick face) is taking over the world and we need to change it. In defense of the female trainer, it's unfortunate that if you say "hi" to a guy, he thinks you like him- guys are idiots. I'm not sure what the answer is, but people need to say "Hello" and "Thank You" more, and most guys need to stop being perverts.

In 2016, I attended a Glute Seminar from Bret Contreras. I paid $400 to see him talk about the glutes- it was glorious! Don't tell me you're passionate about fitness until you see him or Todd Durkin speak- you don't have the right to use the word passion in the same sentence as those two legends. After I got home, I sent Bret a gift card to Amazon as a, "Thank You for your time." He replied by saying in his 17+ years of training, no one has ever done that and wanted to know how he could help me. I didn't send the card with the expectation of something in return, I sent it because my parents raised a good man. Golden rule: Do onto others as you would expect to do upon you. A thank you, a smile, picking up a piece of trash, holding the door, and buying someone a cup of coffee goes a long way. Change the world by helping one person at a time.

7. Three people everyone should follow:

Everyone mentioned in this book (expect Jillian Michaels)

Dr. William Kraemer (My #1 Man crush of all time), Gary Vaynerchuk (Business entrepreneurship), Drunken Humor (sometimes we just gotta laugh at how stupid we can be.)

RESOURCES

By the time this eBook is finished, I will have posted an article on the top ten books / DVD's that all beginning trainers should read. It'll be more in-depth than the following list:

Ignite the Fire by Goodman

Low Back Disorders AND Back Mechanic by McGill

Functional Stability Training by Cressey & Reinold

Alan Aragon's Research Review (monthly)

Strength & Conditioning Research (Contreras & Beardsley) & MASS—Monthly Applications in Strength Sport by Stronger by Science.

Pain by Moseley (DVD)

Hypertophy by Dr. Schoenfeld

Easy Strength by Dan John & Pavel

Precision Nutrition /ISSN by Berardi/Antonio

Science and Practice of Strength Training by Zatsiorsky & Kraemer

10A *The New Rules of Lifting* (Guys, read the girls version.; girls, read the guy's version) by Luo Schuler

Non-Text Books:

So Good They Can't Ignore You by Cal Newport

How to Win Friends and Influence People by Dale Carnegie

Tipping Point by Malcom Gladwell

Never Eat Alone by Keith Ferrazzi

The Power of Habit by Charles Duhigg

Shoe Dog by Phil Knight

Cowboy Ethics by James P. Owen

The Giving Tree by Shel Silverstein

Elon Musk: Tesla, SpaceX, and the Quest for a Fantastic Future Ashlee Vance

Make Your Bed by Admiral William H. McRaven

Shoe Dog? If you haven't realized this by now, you've just entered the world of business, and the product is you. You need to accept and get over the fact that you'll be constantly involved in sales. Within the business world is rejection— get used to it. The only way to get better is practice and learning from your mistakes. As the author of Shoe Dog Phil Knight, says, "Business is war without bullets." Do you want to eat this month? Pay rent? Be able to afford the luxuries of greedy Americans—cars, handbags, Lululemon? If the answer is yes, you better get out there and let the world know how awesome you are. It all starts by changing the mind and body of one person. You cannot grow a garden overnight. It takes time, water, sunlight, and the perfect environment. The same goes with personal training. You will not grow a book of business overnight. Focus on how you can help one person at a time, get up after you've been knocked down, and maintain a positive fucking mindset.

ACKNOWLEDGEMENTS AND PARTING THOUGHTS

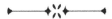

Thank you for taking the time to read *How to Be a Successful Personal Trainer*. I sent over 50 emails and text messages to an equal number of women and men. I understand people are busy; I have no hard feelings to those who didn't respond. People are busy and I can only imagine how many emails top coaches and trainers receive. Thank you to everyone who helped by contributing to this eBook.

You're the future of the training world. Listen to the words from these very successful trainers and remember why you wanted to become a personal trainer in the first place. HELP NICK and implement as many of the keys to be successful as you can. Most personal trainers get certified and stop learning. I challenge you to be significant; don't follow the masses. If you follow blindly and not evolve, you won't make it. I've been a hiring manager and currently manage ten trainers. I wouldn't hire a personal trainer who only has a certification; GO TO SCHOOL AND GET AN INTERNSHIP! Understanding human movement begins in the classroom. As Dean Somerset says, "Watch, observe, try, fail, reassess, try again, find what works, improve that, find stuff you suck at, improve those, repeat." Make your mind right, as Todd Durkin says. If the gym environment doesn't work for you, that's ok, but don't give up after a month. Be creative and persistent like Kellie was—find your passion within the industry. Think and practice like Dan John does. Read anatomy textbooks Like Dr. Rusin says. Don't hop on bandwagons, or any BOSU balls, for that manner, like Tim Henrique says. Do an internship like Ben Bruno says. Give back and don't be an asshole like Tony Gentilcore says. *At the end of the day, THIS IS the right career choice if you focus on helping other people, continue your education, work hard, and as Mr. Charles Staley and I say, SHOW UP!*

Interested in going to school to become a personal trainer? Enroll at the Show Up Fitness Personal Training Academy in Santa Monica.

Show Up Fitness Personal Training Academy in Santa Monica, CA, is a four-month PT school in which you'll learn anatomy, physiology, biomechanics, nutrition, and how to be a successful business trainer. The Academy teaches you to pass the NASM, NSCA, and/or ACSM certifications, but more importantly, allows you to do an internship training a variety of clients. The course is over 300 hours long, with over 200 hours of interning and applied workouts. Oh yeah, and you'll also get into amazing shape while you go to school.

What Separates Show Up Fitness Academy from Other PT schools?

The Show Up Fitness Academy has a Board of Education with top trainers, PhD's, and doctors, along with a four-month internship. Chris Hitchko has graduated over 700-personal trainers and knows the formula to become successful in the fitness industry. Throughout his twelve-year tenure, he's collaborated with top trainers, professors, nutritionists, and doctors, which allowed him to develop a Board of Education to make sure the material and scientific information is up-to-date.

The Show Up Fitness Personal Training Academy Board of Education: Professor Jason Cholewa, PhD Exercise Science, Coastal Carolina; Layne Norton, PhD Nutritional Sciences, University of Illinois; John Rusin, Doctorate in Physical Therapy; Dean Somerset, CSCS; Dr. Chris Perry, MD; Joel Seedman, PhD, University of Georgia.

While attending the Academy, you'll have numerous opportunities to intern and train a variety clients at Show Up Fitness Santa Monica. Upon approval, you can begin training clients and teaching classes. Other training schools try to sell you on "hands on experience"- this means you get to train other students. How the hell are you supposed to gain experience by training someone else who's currently enrolled to become a personal trainer? At the Academy, you'll train paying clients and get an opportunity to help coach athletes at Santa Monica High School. When you graduate, you'll be able to add a four-month internship to your resume. Additionally, there will be opportunities to meet with managers at Equinox, Crunch, Velocity, and other hiring gyms. You'll learn about the everyday life of a trainer, can ask managers questions, and potentially set up future interviews. Chris will teach you how to run a successful personal training company, how to ace an interview, the best ways to get new clients, how to draw up a business plan, SWOT goals, and resume development. If you want to be a successful personal trainer, you need to have confidence in your product. Show Up Fitness Academy will help you become the best personal trainer. The choice is simple, you need to SHOW UP.

Pyramid of Success for weight loss, strength training, performance, and LIFE! If you want to learn more about STD's, Energy Balance, and Winning the Week, you'll need to go to the Show Up Fitness Academy ;-)

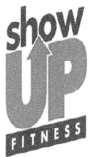

PYRAMID OF
SUCCESS

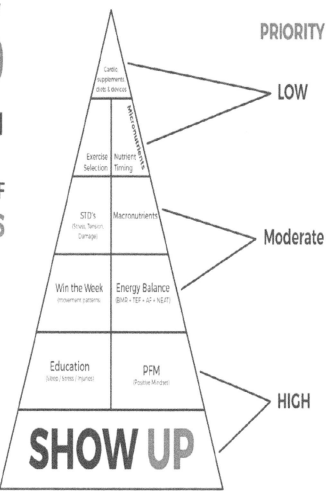

PRIORITY

LOW

Cardio,
supplements,
diets & devices

Micronutrients

Exercise
Selection

Nutrient
Timing

STD's
(Stress, Tension,
Damage)

Macronutrients

Moderate

Win the Week
(movement patterns)

Energy Balance
(BMR + TEF + AF + NEAT)

Education
(Sleep / Stress / Injuries)

PFM
(Positive Mindset)

HIGH

SHOW UP

Made in United States
North Haven, CT
29 June 2023

38377165R00049